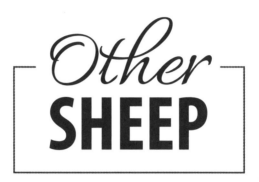

Arnold H. Schroeder

NORTHWESTERN PUBLISHING HOUSE
Milwaukee, Wisconsin

Cover Photo: Shutterstock
Art Director: Karen Knutson
Designer: Paula Clemons

REV. ARNOLD H. SCHROEDER
UPDATED AND REPRINTED *OTHER SHEEP*
NORTHWESTERN PUBLISHING HOUSE
Milwaukee, Wisconsin
Prepared under the auspices of the Commission on Christian Literature, Wisconsin Evangelical Lutheran Synod

Library of Congress Catalog Card Number: 81-80055
Northwestern Publishing House
1250 N. 113th St., Milwaukee, WI 53226-3284
www.nph.net
© 1981 by Northwestern Publishing House. All rights reserved
Published 1981, Revised 2013
Printed in the United States of America
ISBN 978-0-8100-0140-4
ISBN 978-0-8100-2753-4 (e-book)

Institutional Ministries has been richly blessed by the Almighty God for over 113 years. The ministry continues to serve those who cannot come to us, the institutionalized and often members of their families as well.

In thanks to God and in recognition of his blessings, the ministry is pleased to once again make available the book, *Other Sheep*, by Pastor Arnold Schroeder. Chaplain Schroeder was the first full-time institutional missionary in the Wisconsin Evangelical Lutheran Synod. He faithfully served Institutional Ministries on a full-time basis for 40 years, 1938–1978. He wrote the original *OTHER SHEEP* book in 1981. It was published by Northwestern Publishing House, and the original is no longer available in print. Pastor Schroeder was called home to heaven on January 15, 1993.

With the permission of Northwestern Publishing House and with the assistance of Arnold Schroeder's family, WLIM is pleased to offer this new edition of *OTHER SHEEP*. Quotations from Scripture have been updated from the King James translation and a few other edits have been made. We think you will enjoy reading about the many interesting visits Pastor Schroeder shared in his book.

Gospel-based ministry to the institutionalized and their families has not changed in 113 years; the institutionalized continue to need the message of the Savior's love and forgiveness, ours by grace though faith.

May God's blessings continue to rest upon Institutional Ministries and the thousands of people faithfully served with God's Word.

We hope you enjoy reading about sharing the Savior with those in institutions and with the members of their families in *OTHER SHEEP*.

The Board and Staff of Wisconsin Lutheran Institutional Ministries
2323 North Mayfair Road, Suite 480
Wauwatosa, WI 53226
414-259-4370
WLIM @WLIM.net
www.wlim.net

*To my faithful and busy wife who has shared my ministry in
every way, especially by her dedication, encouragements,
and personal services to our Lord's other sheep.*

CONTENTS

I have other sheep that are not of this sheep pen.
I must bring them also. They too will listen to my voice,
and there shall be one flock and one shepherd.

John 10:16

INTRODUCTION

As America entered the twentieth century, Milwaukee Lutherans of the now defunct Synodical Conference became interested in the spiritual welfare of people who were separated from normal church and congregational activities because of poverty, illness, homelessness, imprisonment, and other situations of dependency. Since most hospitals and large special care homes were located in metropolitan areas, four major cities became centers of institutional mission work. Milwaukee was one of them.

Usually the dependent ones were separated from their homes and churches by a considerable distance. Institutions that could provide care for them were located on the outskirts of the city. Before the common use of the automobile and adequate public transport, frequent contact with residents was difficult and sometimes impossible.

Milwaukee in large part was populated by immigrant Lutherans from across the Atlantic, and so it also had large numbers of institutionalized Lutherans. It was easy to lose track of them and forget them once they were confined to a hospital or home quite distant from the family and old friends.

In the late 1890s Pastor William Rader, of St. John's in Wauwatosa, became deeply involved and concerned when on a Sunday afternoon during his exercise walk he passed a large and imposing structure with the inscription on its gates: POOR FARM. (Later it was renamed: COUNTY INFIRMARY.) He was curious. Who lived in such a place, and what did they do?

Quickly retracing his steps, he walked the long block that led to the office where, after proper introduction and an explanation for his curiosity, he soon learned that there were hundreds of people living there. He was also informed that the large 100-bed wards housed many Lutherans, not a few of whom seldom if ever had a visitor call.

By special permission Pastor Rader walked through one or two wards on the first floor. There he talked with a number of residents who appeared to be most unhappy with their lot in life. The isolation and deadly daily routine were snuffing out all desire to continue living and planning. To them this was the end of the road.

The sensitive pastor tried to put himself into their position, and his warm heart soon recognized an important opportunity to serve these aged and despairing people with the consolations of an understanding and compassionate God. The desire within him grew. That first visit led to another and then to many more. It was obvious to him that the Great Shepherd had led an undershepherd to a flock of wandering and lost sheep.

And the Shepherd blessed his servant's efforts with promising responses from the residents. In short order he was conducting worship services there every week. The attendance kept increasing. The spirit of the institution was changing remarkably. The seed of the Word was sown, and God was giving a rich harvest. And the pastor was only too happy to continue his work there over and above his parish duties.

As the superintendents of other care facilities on the 1200-acre county grounds met often to discuss their various needs and responsibilities, Pastor Rader's influence in creating a new atmosphere of wholesomeness and contentment at the Poor Farm became an important topic. Soon administrators of other institutions were asking him to visit their charges. As a dedicated pastor, he tried to fulfill as many requests for group and individual visits as he could. But the burdens of a growing congregation and a lack of time were sapping his strength.

Thoroughly convinced that the Lord looked with favor on this mission effort, he called a meeting of all interested pastors and congregations in the area. He explained his work and its fruits to the assembly, and encouraged all present to find ways and means to pursue and promote the new project. The response was excellent! But since most of the pastors were so busy with their own work, they decided that this worthy evangelism effort needed and warranted the services of a full-time missionary to gather in the harvest the Lord was providing from among the large fields of lonely souls.

They set their objectives and formed a corporation. During the ensuing months the corporation sent out eight calls, as it searched for a pastor to pioneer in a church activity known in only three other metropolitan areas of our nation. Eventually Pastor Enno A. Duemling of Detroit accepted the call. He became the first Milwaukee Institutional and City Missionary (Anstalts und Stadtmissionar) in 1901.

Many were the duties and heavy the responsibilities that rested on his compassionate heart, especially when just a few years later the State Prison in Waupun (sixty-five miles away) was added as a station to be served from Milwaukee. Even a young man found the pace killing. So at the time of the twenty-fifth anniversary of Institutional Missions, Pastor John Helmes of Menasha, Wisconsin, was called to and accepted the position of associate pastor. Together the pastors served a field of more than ten large institutions with a population of over 10,000 people. Then, when both pastors were aging beyond their years under heavy assignments, the author of this book was called in 1938 to share a work now firmly established and entrenched in local church life.

For forty-two of his more than forty-six years in the Lutheran ministry the writer has deemed it a special blessing to serve our gracious and long-suffering Lord in a field that grips the heart with the plight of so many of our Master's needy brethren. This call has been carried out at Milwaukee County General Hospital, the Hospital for Mental Diseases or the Asylum for the Chronic Insane (now a combined Mental Health Center), at a tuberculosis sanatorium, at a home for dependent children, at a house of correction or U.S. disciplinary barracks or state prisons and industrial schools, at the U.S. veterans' facilities, at half-way houses, nursing and convalescent homes, and at many another "house of misery." In this work one thing has always been amazing, and that is THE POWER OF GOD'S WORD AND THE SACRAMENTS in turning lives around from hopelessness and despair to faith in God's promises and peace for living.

No medical or surgical means, no psychological techniques or psychiatric treatments, no social correctional policies and practices, no experiments or human reforms can do what God does by his MEANS OF GRACE—heal the hurting heart and soul and deliver it into an eternity of bliss. This has been the experience of an undershepherd who has preached, taught, baptized, communed, counseled, and buried a host of "other sheep" in many crisis situations. During these many years of specialized ministry he has witnessed the tremendous and sometimes unbelievable power of the Word as it brought calm out of chaos, comfort in calamity, peace in turbulence, and a new and powerful life to many a straying sheep that by time and circumstances had long been removed from the security of the flock.

This book is intended solely to exalt a gracious and glorious God, who might well have reserved this privilege for his angels, yet placed it into the hands of sinful men. May Christians everywhere appreciate their priceless heritage as chosen and kept children of God!

All the stories recorded are actual case histories. Though not always exact verbatim accounts, they are true reflections of real people and events hidden away from normal view behind the curtain of institutional missions. Names, of course, have been altered.

A. H. S.

THE SHEPHERD AND HIS SHEEP

After Adam and Eve had plunged the world and every one to be born in it into misery and condemnation by their sins of unbelief and rebellion, that wonderful sensation of security that existed in Eden was gone. And the more the world became populated, the greater became the alienation between God and man. In too many lives there was a misdirection that led only to impotent self-reliance with its uncountable fears and eventual hopelessness. Life became a frantic search for an anchor that would steady the ship of life tossed about in heavy seas.

In God's foreknowledge, however, he fashioned a way to restore security and peace. He would make right what man had made wrong. He would send his Son Jesus, one of the Holy Trinity of Father, Son and Holy Spirit, as a man of flesh and blood like other humans. In a hopeless world he would assure all men of pardon for sin and the gift of eternal life with him in heaven.

He chose the people of Israel as the vehicle by which the God-man would come into the world. Through his word and promises to Israel he would lead his people to the cross of Calvary on which the Redeemer one day would die in full atonement for all sins.

It is interesting to note that God in the Bible selected to use a familiar picture to depict his concerns, his mercies, and his love for fallen mankind. It was the picture of a shepherd deeply involved in looking after the welfare of his sheep, the flock. Something like this his people could understand, because shepherding for many was a part of daily life. And then in his own selected time he would bring the one great Good Shepherd, the Son-Savior, into this hodgepodge on earth, so that never again would man be without an answer for his restlessness. And man's reconciliation with God became history on that first Good Friday on a hill outside the gate of Jerusalem.

The Bible speaks of sheep without a shepherd (Numbers 27:17), of sheep going astray (Deuteronomy 22:1), of sheep stolen (2 Samuel 12:4), of sheep scattered (Ezekiel 34:6), and of lost sheep (Luke 15:4).

How fitting a description of man this is. A sheep is said to be a dumb animal, easily frightened, erring, and wandering away from the flock. It is stubborn and self-willed, insensitive to dangers. It becomes lost and dies—a perfect resemblance of natural man.

To such the Good Shepherd would come to restore order and meaning to life. "The Shepherd of Israel", he was called by David long before he was born (Psalm 80:1). For 4000 years the faithful waited for the first Christmas in Bethlehem.

Suddenly he came! Poor, lowly, humble, he accepted his servant role. But later, established in his ministry, Jesus was a man to be heard. He claimed, "I am the good shepherd. The good shepherd lays down his life for the sheep." (John 10:11). Jesus was the long-awaited One. His words and miracles proved his claim to be true.

Yet to seek and to save the lost was not an easy task. Even the organized religious activities of those days were a hindrance, rather than a help. But Jesus kept his eye on the goal, all the way to the cross and beyond. Patiently and lovingly he kept calling to all: "Come to me."

When he was ready to return home to his throne above, his orders were to evangelize the whole world. Jesus said: "Feed my lambs" and "Take care of my sheep" (John 21:15, 16). The response is recorded especially in the Book of Acts and in the history of the Christian Church throughout the ages.

You and I, professing Christians in a modern age, are the fruits of the Shepherd's labors and sufferings. He has drawn us to himself, enlightened our understanding, and made us unashamed of the gospel, which we recognize as the only power that can bring salvation. Deeply imbedded in our hearts is the assurance that we are HIS SHEEP.

We meet other believers in him. We walk together and talk together. We unite our efforts by forming congregations of like-minded and like-dedicated people to keep on sharing the good news of forgiveness, redemption, and unending life. This is the flock of the Shepherd, the church. In its visible form it is impure and weak because it is made up of sinful humans. Nevertheless, it contains God's elect who will one day be gathered around his throne.

We realize, though, that not all of his sheep live comfortably within the corporate structure of congregational life. Some, our neighbors far and near, are still scattered and wandering, searching for the safety of the Shepherd's fold. Some may be thousands of miles away in Africa, India, Japan, China, or in North and South America. They may be little flocks or large flocks. They may be isolated individuals and families, living apart from the mainstream of life.

These are the OTHER SHEEP Jesus refers to when he says, "I have other sheep that are not of this sheep pen. I must bring them also. They too will listen to my voice, and there shall be one flock and one shepherd." (John 10:16).

This background explains the intensity of our mission efforts throughout the world. In the Wisconsin Evangelical Lutheran Synod we expend millions of dollars annually to gather and feed our Shepherd's sheep, so that when they "walk through the valley of the shadow of death," they shall fear no evil. We want them to know that the Lord is with them; his rod and his staff will sustain and comfort them (Psalm 23).

We also expend large amounts of special monies—compassion gifts, if you will—for institutional mission work. In our nation there are approximately 7000 licensed and approved hospitals and health care centers, including state prisons and other correctional detention centers. Put together, this is a huge flock of more than thirty-three million hidden-away sheep! In every place we should let the gospel call be heard by sick, lost, and erring sheep and lambs.

The soil is most fertile and productive where the miseries of sin are taking their daily toll. Our call is clear: "Repent of your wrongdoing; receive the gift of God's pardon and peace." And many, not all, will respond: "O Lamb of God, I come, I come." The call is heard by means of group worship services, but most opportunely and effectively by visits on a person-to-person basis. Whoever shepherds for Christ in such circumstances quickly forgets the difficulties and deadly routine, the physical drain and the mental fatigue of his labors. He remembers sheep heeding the Good Shepherd's voice, following him, and being happy at entering or returning to the fold.

Most of the sheep the average Christian knows are the brothers and sisters in Christ who gather regularly in the Lord's House around the Word and sacraments. Ordinarily they come from a Christian home, have had the advantage of Christian training in church and school, have heard the Shepherd's voice and followed him. When one of these has strayed and temporarily or permanently left the flock our heart bleeds. We in the family of God suffer while we seek to return the lost one and pray for the wanderer's return.

How happy we are when the Lord answers our prayers through the efforts of an undershepherd! The prodigal son comes home!

TRIALS PRODUCE TESTIMONY

Maury's story is typical of a modern prodigal son. He was born to a Lutheran family in southern Indiana, baptized into the kingdom, and at age fourteen confirmed in his faith before the Lord's altar. His adolescence was, as he later recalled, the happiest time of his life. His church was closely interlaced in his personal affairs.

After graduation from high school he occupied himself with a number of jobs that were of no consequence. And then came the big break. He was employed by a national industry as a salesman, and this position suited him perfectly. He was a very outgoing person, and this was a plus in the many contacts he made with people from all walks of life. Promotion followed promotion, and soon Maury was traveling throughout the Midwest for his firm.

Serious as his intentions were to remain with the church, he found less and less opportunity to worship in his accustomed way. Besides, the influences of customers and business associates were making themselves felt, and these influences were not conducive to the Christian way of living. Without his realizing it, he was withdrawing farther and farther from church, and before he analyzed what was happening to him, he was mired in the slime of materialism and hedonistic pleasures to the point that he no longer needed God to satisfy his inner man. Occasional conscience reminders were quickly muffled. He left the church entirely and seldom gave thought to what he was sacrificing by way of true contentment, peace for a troubled conscience, and good guidance and strength for daily living.

Years rolled by during which he never reflected on these vital things until, broken down in health by his fast pace, he developed a serious lung disease (in those days more often fatal than curable). The months of hospitalization turned into years, and there was no promise of improvement. But that time of his life later proved to be one of great blessing.

As he thought back on his earlier life, especially his youthful days, a "nagging something" made him extremely restless, irritable, and sullen. He felt cheated, and more so as his wife divorced him on the grounds of incompatibility. Oh, how this troubled sheep needed a shepherd! Though his ears had been deafened to the call of the Good Shepherd, an awakening conscience and a series of incidental events brought him to see himself again as a lost sinner in need of a Father's forgiveness and help.

Another man of fine Christian character, a devout Lutheran, shared Maury's room at the sanatorium. When this man read his Bible and devotional books every morning and evening, it was a strong reminder of how important God is for a satisfying existence in days of affliction. The roommate, with but a short time to live, was the picture of a confident and assured man waiting patiently for the day when the Lord would call him out of this vale of tears.

As missionary or "chaplain" in this 650-bed house of misery, I met Maury one day while calling on his roommate. He was most anxious to meet a "man of God" and to empty his heart of so many deep concerns. The loneliness and fear of a sheep that had lost its way was becoming too much for him to bear. There followed a long series of very profitable visits which stressed many Biblical assurances that the Good Shepherd Jesus had come into our world to erase our guilt by atoning for our sins. All the shame of our forgetfulness and indifference was now hidden in his precious blood.

One could sense that the once deaf ears were again opening and listening intently to the call of the Shepherd. Earnestly Maury was trying to find his way back to the security of the fold. After reviewing the fundamental truths, he accepted our invitation to attend the chapel services every Wednesday night and soon became an avid churchgoer. In due time, he joined our group of communicants to whom the personal assurance of the sacrament meant more than we can imagine.

Maury often tried to rationalize his condition, and in so doing he came up with the right answer for his physical suffering: God in his endless love had found a way to bring his sheep back to the security of the family of his sons and daughters!

Sometimes it was hard for Maury to understand God's ways, just as it is for us to follow his thoughts toward us. He might easily have turned away again from his Shepherd as his condition steadily worsened. But he didn't. He clung to the promise that his heavenly Father's ways were ways of peace and not of evil. Still it wasn't at all easy for Maury to suffer pain patiently and watch his life ebbing.

In surgery our patient lost his entire right rib cage, and his heart had to be padded and taped to what was left of his chest. He was now an incurable, chronic invalid who could look ahead to nothing better than a hospital or institutional residence for the remainder of his life. And this happened at about age fifty!

The story doesn't end there. Instead of becoming a disillusioned and bitter man, Maury was asking: "Lord, what will you have me do?" Never did we hear a complaint that the Good Shepherd was ignoring or mistreating his sheep. Rather, in daily repentance and the remembrance of God's love, he found strength and courage to endure. And little did he realize or imagine the plans his Shepherd had for him, but as they slowly developed he found happiness and peace. Amazing things were in the

TAKE HEED!

If you poison the well, many people will lose their life as they drink of the polluted water. Satan is well aware of this basic truth. When he wants to detour many souls to hell, he will try to poison the source of their spiritual food and drink. In church life, this means that when he succeeds in misleading an undershepherd, he begins to count numberless victims who have been following that shepherd or have been influenced by his leadership.

Vocational and professional workers in the church—undershepherds if you will—are not guaranteed immunity against the wiles of the devil. In fact, in many ways they may become targets of severe temptations in connection with their work in the kingdom. We are not surprised, except for feeling the shame, that occasionally we hear of and meet a pastor or teacher who has been through the mill of the Evil One and victimized by his sweet wiles.

Pastors may be tempted to immorality by an unscrupulous woman in the congregation. Teachers must constantly practice self-discipline in intimate contacts with children in their classes. And by the very nature of their work, wanting to sympathize and to help, they may unwittingly be led into a trap of sin from which there is no easy exit. Our heart goes out to them. In our contacts with fallen leaders of the church we have learned that the road back is never an easy one. The difficulties are multiplied just because of the former honored position of the fallen. When the full impact of their sin is realized and the inevitable consequences must be faced squarely, the results are pitiful to behold.

Whether it is in a psychiatric hospital or in a prison, when you find a fallen shepherd, you know that the return to normalcy will be difficult and long in coming. Satan, who initiated the fall, has powerful tools at his disposal, the most powerful being the Word of God! That very gospel of pardon and hope which the shepherds preached and taught is now thrown before them as a stumbling block in their quest for peace. How quick the devil is in his unholy attempt to convince a professing Christian, turned public sinner, that his sin is unpardonable because it was committed in spite of better knowledge. Imagine if you can his glee as he feeds the feelings of self-humiliation and disgrace and fans the fires of fear in him who once declared the unconditional pardon of God for every penitent!

Though God's forgiveness is free and limitless, self-forgiveness is difficult. Most miserable are the men, so ashamed and sorrowful, who try with all their might to cling to assurances of God's rich forgiveness, and are at the same time tormented by their self-condemnation and the horrendous thought of returning one day to face the people who once respected them so highly as ambassadors of the gospel. The thundering "you shall not!" of the Law tends to drive them into deep depression. In one case it took six months before a troubled young man felt worthy to receive the sacrament. God's power overcame Satan's trickery.

Persistent reminders of the Good Shepherd and his ways with us mortals have their effect in time, under God. What relief and joy the offender experiences when the Spirit strengthens his faith! And what a new depth of understanding of love follows that daily digging in the furrows of Scripture: that unstoppable praying and pleading; that blessedness of the Savior's body and blood in Holy Communion.

Hopelessness has a way of disappearing when God is close at hand. The Shepherd in his tender mercies continues to supply the power to smile through tears and to restore his sheep to useful occupations; yes, possibly to make him a greater blessing to the kingdom in days to come.

I met one of these fallen ones a few months ago—in a restaurant, over a cup of coffee. He was spiritually well and sound, thanks to the power that saves—God's eternal Word.

A FAMILY IN TROUBLE

St. Paul warned the disciples: "I know that after I leave, savage wolves will come in among you and will not spare the flock." (Acts 20:29) He was repeating a caution Jesus had mentioned (Matthew 10:16): "I am sending you out like sheep among wolves." And the chief destroyer and enemy is always the devil.

What has been said before about the devil attacking professional church leaders must be said also of lay leaders in congregations. Chop at the roots, and hopefully the tree will die. Satan will use every trick in his bag to give the church's enemies an excuse to point fingers at the family of God. If he can lead a leader into disgraceful conduct and public sin and shame, he can win more to his side and lead them to destruction.

I well remember a council member of an upstate church. He was the church treasurer, who under great stress lost his sense of direction and dedication. During the last World War he worked many hours of overtime every day, and his wife helped with the family finances by working the night shift. Earnings were excellent; the future looked rosy. But what a life! They seldom saw each other long enough for conversation, and the children in the family seldom saw their parents. More often than not, when the children went to church, they went alone. Dad and Mother were working. Supervision and management of the family were left to chance.

What a prime time for Satan to throw temptation after temptation before this family! And he did! The father began to drink heavily "to relax from the grind," while the mother looked for outside companionship during her free hours. There was little if any concern for the children growing up. The parents were enjoying their new style of free and easy living. More and more, and subtly, God was left out of the picture.

And then it happened! They had to learn the hard way that God is not mocked. What one sows brings a crop that must be reaped. One day the father came home in a stuporous condition and, seeing his thirteen-year-old daughter in scanty attire, was overcome by unchaste desires. He forced his own daughter into an immoral act. She reported this to the police; the father was arrested, tried in court, and promptly sent to prison. A few months later the daughter was sent to a home for unwed mothers in a distant city. Both became my charges at the request of their pastor.

What a wagging of tongues followed in the home town! Satan pulled out all the stops as people pointed fingers at the church and its members. The deriders of our Savior had their inning, and they made the most of it. We couldn't deny the facts: a part of the flock had been invaded and driven out of the fold. We had a smutty and sensitive situation to deal with. What can one say?

We must remember that the Good Shepherd neither slumbers nor sleeps as he watches his flock, even from some distance. Both of the principals involved in this story acknowledged their disgraceful conduct as a serious offense against God, and both were willing to listen to the Shepherd's voice. There was much sobbing, deep and bitter remorse as both passed through the throes of sincere repentance. The only thing that really counted now was not society's satisfaction for the crime, but Christ's glorious promise: "Then neither do I condemn you. Go now and leave your life of sin," (John 8:11).

At the same time that we were ministering to the father in prison, we were instructing, comforting, and helping direct the spiritual rehabilitation of the daughter in her strange surroundings. Years later the whole family was reunited and walked with blessing in close proximity with the Shepherd, praying and working that never again would they become easy prey for him who walks about as a roaring lion, seeking whom he may devour.

The whole sad story turned out to be a blessing in disguise for the family, for the church, and for the community. The malicious barbs aimed at the church were warded off by the renewed dedication of this family that had passed through the fires of purification. Some former scoffers too were attracted.

THE WAY OF THE TRANSGRESSOR

Everyone in our community was stunned when the headline in the newspaper screamed out in bold letters: YOUTH SHOOTS MOTHER, BROTHER, SISTER. The youth was from one of our churches and known to many. But now he stood before the world as a ruthless murderer! And he was still in his teens.

In a fit of rage because he was denied the use of the family car, he ran to his room, loaded his gun, and came back downstairs to take revenge on his mother by shooting her! The preteen sister scrambled under the bed to get out of the way; he shot her. The little brother ran toward the phone to call the police; he shot him too. Blind passion sent three souls to eternity in a matter of just a few minutes.

Pete had all the advantages of a sheep of the flock. From early childhood his mother had taught him to know the Shepherd. Pete walked with him through Christian day school, heard more of him in high school training, and was under his influence in regular worship and Communion attendance. There was real promise of many years of blessings ahead.

Sometimes, however, the Good Shepherd's ways were too dull and restricting for a youth growing up in the big city. The sheep began to look around for other companionship, and he found it among sheep of other folds and other shepherds. They seemed to have much more freedom from self-discipline, and this was a strong attraction. Though the spirit had not lost its willingness to abide by the Shepherd, yet the flesh became weaker and weaker.

Then came that horrible evening that Pete will never forget to his dying day. He was out for fun, but his mother stood in the way. He was disappointed, then angry, then furious. Losing all control of sense and reason, he shed his family's blood! How forcefully we are reminded of the warning of James: "When tempted, no one should say, 'God is tempting me.' For God cannot be tempted by evil, nor does he tempt anyone; but each person is tempted when they are dragged away by their own evil desire and enticed. Then, after desire has conceived, it gives birth to sin; and sin, when it is full-grown, gives birth to death" (James 1:13-15).

Pete was sent to prison on a life term, and his search for freedom was over. There was no freedom, only regimentation, rules, routines. There were taunters and deriders to rub elbows with daily. Unlike his home, there was no room of his own, only a small cell with iron doors. There was no comfortable bed, made and kept clean by a loving mother, only a wall-hanging steel frame with a thin mattress. There was no separate bathroom with shower and tub and clean fluffy towels, only a basin and a toilet attached to the bare plaster wall. Signals summoned the men to line up in formation for meals or occasional recreation time. The food was wholesome, but institutional and predictable, day by day. Hundreds of men ate together in silence in the huge dining room three times each day. And when the lights went out in mid-evening there were the endless hours of darkness—and memories! What a life!

The darkness of night was but a reflection of the darkness and ignorance of sin and degradation. What can possibly pierce it and provide light for our path and a lamp for our way? Only the powerful Word of God; mark it well!

Pete rediscovered that. For some time he was too ashamed to think about his Lord, too timid to knock at God's door. But the Good Shepherd had not forgotten nor forsaken this disgraced sheep. His voice was to be heard also behind prison walls. The young man listened to it in our chapel services, and it revived and recovered a faith that had worn thin.

In private visits and in our group meetings the Holy Spirit invaded his thinking: not with the "you must" of the Commandments, but with the "God did" of the healing gospel. "If we confess our sins, he is faithful and just and will forgive us our sins and purify us from all unrighteousness." (1 John 1:9). Pete's heart was good soil for such seeding, and the sunshine of grace brought good fruits. Strengthened by Word and sacrament, Pete began to plan the rebuilding of his broken life. Physically, emotionally, and spiritually he matured rapidly, and the Shepherd's profound love and evidences of his compassionate care became the foundation for the future. Without that Savior, those long months and longer years behind prison walls might easily have led to utter shipwreck.

When the time for release on parole came many years later, Pete determined to walk the path of his Shepherd Savior. He went to church in spite of the embarrassment this caused at times; he occupied his time by working hard; he met a good companion and married her. Through it all he struggled as best he could to forget the ugly past, especially three graves in a nearby cemetery.

One afternoon, as I was driving to the hospital for calls, a lightweight truck followed closely. Over the space of several blocks the driver of the truck repeatedly, insistently sounded his horn. In irritation I pulled to the curb, to let him pass, only to notice through the mirror that the truck came to a stop right behind me. A man jumped out and approached my car. His hand was outstretched in warm greeting. It was my friend Pete from prison!

Can you imagine the expressions of joy from both of us? Briefly we reminisced over bygone years and reviewed happenings since then. We agreed that the love and mercy of our Savior-God made so true his promise: "And we know that in all things God works for the good of those who love him, who have been called according to his purpose." (Romans 8:28)

From disgraced sinner to exalted saint. How impossible is man's frantic pursuit of achievement! But how possible and real for him who made us, and in whom we live and move and have our being!

If Pete could address us today, I'm sure that among the other things he might have to say would be an urgent appeal to "Watch and pray so that you will not fall into temptation. The spirit is willing, but the flesh is weak" (Matthew 26:41).

PANIC PACIFIED

Being "on call" as a hospital pastor sometimes puts one on a veritable merry-go-round of activity. At our large General Hospital we were expected to be ready twenty-four hours per day to respond to all kinds of emergencies and also to make ward rounds to search out the "Lutherans" admitted for care.

In a large city there are, of course, many emergencies occurring every day. People are victims of serious traffic accidents, or they suddenly become violently ill, or an injured or diseased organ of the body may demand immediate surgical attention. It was the custom and order in our hospital to refer all such cases to the chaplaincy department, and scarcely a day passed in which we were not summoned several times to make a special emergency call.

In the space of just a few months we had a series of major train and transit crashes which brought scores of people (50 - 75 - 110) into and through the emergency rooms and trauma center to whatever ward beds were available. The hospital had a well-planned "disaster program" by which all available off-duty help was summoned immediately to assist in caring for the injured. And the chaplains were included in the program. They were called to look after the spiritual needs of the critical cases. (Sadly we must report that this ideal plan is now swiftly disappearing because of the "Science is God" philosophy adopted by too many of our modern health care institutions.)

How well I remember the time we had two major accidents, both caused by derailments of rapid transit trains. They were being phased out of the picture of mass transportation, and our local system drew attention from many railroad buffs throughout the nation. Large gatherings of fans were staged and, of course, the folks were taken for a final ride on an "interurban" as a feature of the convention. On one such occasion the hobbyists were treated to their thrilling trip late one afternoon. There was gaiety and excitement galore as the men, women, and little children, whole families, set out from the terminal for a fifteen mile round trip. Maybe it was due to improperly maintained tracks, maybe to some mechanical failure, but the accident was quick and disastrous. Several cars were thrown off the tracks, and great was the wreckage. About fifty riders were rushed to our hospital by whatever means of transit could be found. Many were badly mangled; some appeared to be dying. As I went from bed to bed (and some were lined up in the corridors), I came upon a woman in great distress. She had suffered a skull fracture, fractures of arms and legs, and many painful bruises and abrasions. More distressing to her was the agony of not knowing what had happened to her husband and baby; both had been next to her in the seat before the crash. She had no way of knowing where they might be, whether or not they had been hurt badly, possibly had even been fatally injured.

From our conversation after she regained consciousness I learned that she was a well-informed and active Lutheran from Illinois. And how grateful she was to have a pastor at her side to guide her thinking toward the Great Physician who is never overpowered by accidental happenings in his children's lives. The Word and prayer and sacrament increased her hope and confidence.

But her deep concerns about the family were surely understandable. So, as soon as we could, we began checking the casualty lists and the routing of those who had been in the crash. A few hours later we were able to return to the woman's room with good news. The husband had been taken to another hospital; his injuries were not too serious and would keep him confined for no more than a week or so. The baby, found at the scene lying under a seat cushion, was somewhat upset but otherwise in good condition—and he was on another floor of our hospital! A nurse later brought him to his mother's room just to reassure her that the child was alive and well. Panic had been turned to pleasure in the midst of great pain.

The mother spent many weeks in her bed. Fractures were attended to, surgery was performed, and a long period of rehabilitation was prescribed. For a long time she was unable to take the risk of being transferred to a hospital in her home town. And during those weeks I saw her almost daily as she thirstily drank of the water of life and prayed so fervently for release from these "evil" days. So often we spoke of God's marvelous ways with his sheep, even when for the moment those ways were hard to understand and accept. But there was never a doubt in her mind about God's rightness and goodness in dealing with undeserving sinners. She trusted with all her heart. She lived under her Shepherd's tender care, particularly when emotions and sentiments filled her eyes with tears.

One Sunday morning after the chapel service I went to her room to share with her the thoughts of the sermon, the story of Jacob's ladder at Bethel. Her eyes began to shine as she let her thoughts dwell on Jacob's precarious trip across wastelands to an uncertain reception at Laban's home. The nights spent all alone in faraway places, the loneliness, and the fears—all seemed so much like her own present situation. And then she thought about the ladder he saw in his dream: angels ascending and descending. She applied the lesson to herself saying, "My prayers and yours are being carried by the angels up the ladder to our Lord's throne. He knows exactly how to answer them, and he sends his good answers via the angels who encamp around my bed!" She lived daily in that power.

For a long time after her trying hospital experience this woman and her husband would call by phone as they passed through our city on their way to the north woods. Always, there was that sincere expression of thanks for having kept the Shepherd near, as a troubled and trembling sheep was battling its way back to health and happiness.

We close this chapter with the significant words of the hymn:

> *Oh, blest the house, whate'er befall,*
> *Where Jesus Christ is all in all!*
> *A home that is not wholly his—*
> *How sad and poor and dark it is!*
>
> *Oh, blest that house where faith you find*
> *And all within have set their mind*
> *To trust their God and serve him still*
> *And do in all his holy will! (CW #506: 1–2)*

SCATTERED AND WANDERING SHEEP

All through his earthly life Jesus was dwelling on the purpose of his advent in time. As one of the Holy Trinity that planned our salvation he was fully conscious of the demands the Messiah-role would make on him, and he willingly consented to fulfill them. He knew there would be enmity followed by the cross. He would die that we might live.

It was difficult for the disciples to grasp this. In spite of the fact that Jesus tried by word and deed to imbed understanding in them, so that the work of his church could go on after he returned to heaven's throne, they were so slow to perceive. Possibly it was the security of his daily presence that pulled down the shades before their insight. At any rate, until the very end he continued his efforts to enlighten them.

On that gruesome night before his death, as they walked from the upper room over the Kidron to Gethsemane, he reminded them with a quote from the prophet Zechariah: "I will strike the shepherd, and the sheep of the flock will be scattered." (Matthew 26:31).

Little did anyone that night think of the expansive meaning of those words for the centuries to follow. Yet instinctively and perhaps somewhat automatically they lived and worked in such manner as to prove the truth of the Savior's words. They began to search everywhere for friends of the crucified Christ. No cost was too expensive, no self-denial or self-sacrifice too deterring. The searching and finding of his sheep was the one and all of their existing. They were indeed working out the beautiful prophecy of Ezekiel concerning God's intent to rescue the perishing (Ezekiel 34).

They approached Jews and gentiles alike, for only through the one Shepherd could any human being find his way back to God. With all their heart they believed his word: Jesus answered, "I am the way and the truth and the life. No one comes to the Father except through me" (John 14:6).

As was to be expected, and in keeping with Jesus' own plans, they first made their approach and appeal to their kinsmen, the Jews. There was a church and a depth of religiousness, centering about the great Temple in Jerusalem. There were various "denominations" such as the Pharisees, the Sadducees, and the Essenes. The meaningful traditions of their proud heritage were observed with fanfare and fervor. But something was lacking, and the humble fishermen, Peter and James and John and all the rest, had learned by the grace of God to put the finger on the trouble spot: Religion in their day had blinded itself to the true Light, Jesus the Messiah.

Recorded clearly in the Gospels and Acts is the story of Jesus' many attempts to right the ship, sometimes working independently, but mostly using the disciples to teach, warn, exhort, admonish, and plead with the chosen race. At times also in righteous anger he berated and threatened, but we find no record of mass conversions, except at Pentecost. Instead there was growing hatred and bitterness that climaxed in the cross.

We might say, by comparison with our day, that there was ignorance, mind blocking, and much difficult adjustment between Judaism and Christianity. Yet, one by one, Jesus had the satisfaction of seeing his church grow. Though the process was long and tedious, scattered and wandering sheep were hearing his voice and were being restored to the flock. The great push, of course, came from the gentile world, especially after God's chosen vessel Paul began his missionary journeys in the Mediterranean regions.

Are there Jewish Christians today? Some Christian leaders would be slow to answer that question. Jewish traditionalism is exceedingly strong, and national pride (as displayed in the Zionist movement) sets barricades on the way to him who is "the Way." Yet we know that there are Christian Jews, without trying to estimate the number. In one to one contacts and more often than not in the institutional field, we see the gospel of Christ crucified shine from the heart and in the life of a Jewish person.

JESUS THE MESSIAH

Becky, a Jewess of fine family tradition, was confined to her bed in a hospital for more than a year. We knew her quite well after a time, having stopped many times at her door to exchange pleasantries with her. It was somewhat of a surprise, though, when one day she asked that I step into the room and close the door behind me. You could tell immediately that something heavy was resting on her mind; she wasn't her usual cheerful self. She seemed so anxious to talk. We did. There were questions, as though she were probing my knowledge and veracity in religious matters. But then the surprise: "Chaplain, would you please get me a New Testament of the Scriptures?" I promised that I would, and then asked her what had created the interest to ask for the story of the Messiah-Jesus, who was still taboo among her people as Savior and Lord. She replied: "Oh, I believe that Jesus is God's Son. Man cannot do the things he did like turning water into wine at the happy wedding in Cana. I have been listening to your chapel broadcasts every week (they were channeled to every bed) and have found them very interesting. I love the stories about Jesus and my people, and I believe them."

We were happy to provide her with the Testament, and future visits showed that she spent many hours with it and read it with understanding and faith. Suddenly one day she became critically ill and at her request I was summoned to her bedside. Her plea was simple: "Tell me again that Jesus is my Shepherd and Savior, I want the confidence David had in Psalm 23. I will see him soon."

Her other request was very personal, and understandable: "If anyone should speak with you about it, please don't tell them, especially my relatives, that I am a Christian. They would ignore me, not even bury me." (Her immediate family was strongly orthodox, and we honored her concerns.) Important in the whole case was only one thing: A wandering sheep of the house of Israel had in God's own ways been led back to the sheepfold!

25

Recalling this incident, I was reminded of another; that of a Spanish-Jew who was serving time in prison. He became quite friendly with a man who was attending our instruction course and, among other things, they occasionally got into some heated discussions and arguments on the subject of religion. This led him to attend our chapel worship and later also our class.

In an interview he told me that his mother was a Jewess, his father of Spanish descent. He had lived in five different states, mostly in Colorado, where he had found temporary employment as he was "bumming" his way around the country. He had lost contact with home and family through his meanderings and now was all alone in the world. While in our state he had become inebriated one night and, short of funds, had strong-armed someone and taken his wallet. He was arrested, tried, found guilty, and sent to prison.

We had to give him credit for wanting to do something about making a fresh start in life so that he might become a respectable person. Too often this is only a sham battle in a chronic offender. But Felix was sincere. He walked down every avenue of the past looking for the mistakes that had brought him to his present unhappy home.

In his searching there came back to mind many things his mother had tried to teach him about God. He knew that there is a God and that man is responsible before him for his actions. Yet Felix had felt that as long as God wasn't making his presence felt in man's life, there was no cause for worry or a change of direction. Moreover, he was puzzled as he remembered also the violent arguments in his home in his childhood days. These occurred when the father would insist that the family go to his Catholic church. Felix talked with his father many times about the differences in religion, but the answers to his questions tended only to confuse him more than before.

Could it be that there are false religions and a true religion? If so, how does one separate the good from the bad? With that beginning and with his acceptance of the Bible (both the Old and New Testaments) he was ready to read, listen, and learn. The seeds of knowledge and faith were sown by the Holy

Spirit, and they grew into a healthy sapling. About eighteen months later the young man was ready to confess before everyone that "Christ Jesus came into the world to save sinners—of whom I am the worst" (1 Timothy 1:15). It was a happy Confirmation Day! "I BELIEVE IN JESUS."

Likewise do I remember meeting another Jewess, Cecilia, an aged and ill woman who was making her home at the infirmary. She had become bedridden and was now a patient in the large sick ward.

While ministering to one of our very ill old saints I spoke about that wonderful Savior who loved us with an everlasting love, died to remove the curse of sin and death from us, and held in reserve for us a future of glory with him in heaven. Our meditation was centered in what we call "the gospel in a nutshell" from John 3:16: "For God so loved the world that he gave his one and only Son, that whoever believes in him shall not perish but have eternal life." And we prayed that God would fulfill his promise and let his good will be done in what remained of the life of this sheep of his fold.

I felt a hand tapping weakly at my back. (There were 120 beds in this ward and the space between them was minimal. A patient with outstretched arm could almost touch the next bed.) When I turned around Cecilia was smiling and wanted to say something. She knew I was "a minister from the church" who came through the ward often to talk to the people, so I might be interested in what she had to say. "I am of the Jewish faith, but I believe in Jesus."

This could, under varied circumstances, mean many things, good and bad. But as I took the time to probe a bit, asking her pointed questions about the Messiah, I found her confession to be right and genuine. She did believe in Jesus, though her knowledge of him was sketchy.

At just this time we were making a change in our staff schedule of assignments, and so I couldn't pursue Cecilia's instruction. We soon saw, however, that the Lord of the church uses insignificant happenings, like a change in staff, for his own purposes. Our new coworker was much enthused and encouraged by his first contact in institutional mission work. That contact was Cecilia, whose soul proved to be fertile soil for the gospel. He enjoyed instructing her in the truths of Scripture and in due time confirmed her. It helped immeasurably in warming his heart for service to individual scattered and wandering sheep.

A VARIED FLOCK

Somewhat unusual also is the case of a Jewish man who came to us "by accident." Our first meeting was in a mental health facility where he had been sent for some minor adjustments in his thinking apparatus.

One Sunday morning he wandered into the chapel, and since our regular organist was unable to be with us, he volunteered to play the piano for the hymn singing. After the service we thanked him and engaged him in conversation. He was from a convalescent home, which was church related, and he had taken an interest in Lutheran teaching and worship. That is why he had come to the services that morning; he understood they were to be Lutheran.

He was quite an intelligent conversationalist, and we spent much time with him whenever we were visiting on his ward. In spite of the fact that he was not at all ready to commit himself to an acceptance of Christ as Savior, one could sense that he was more than "nibbling at the bait." Since music was his forte, we spoke frequently about our hymns and the Bible background for their words. This appealed to him, and he spent much time studying the hymnal.

On release from this institution, he was transferred to a large nursing home where, fortunately, we also had the privilege of conducting services. He was happy and honored to be asked to play the organ in chapel, and to the best of our knowledge, he is still serving the Lord in his own way at this place many years later.

Will we meet this wandering sheep in heaven? Only God knows. But the seeds of life have been planted and nourished, and we dare hope that his soul will be in the harvest.

RECOGNIZING THE SHEPHERD'S VOICE

The disciples of the Lord recognized no racial barriers. They were ready to share their treasure of truth with anyone anywhere. And that is as it should be. Twenty centuries later the master's modern disciples surely will want to follow in his steps and preach the gospel to every creature. With more than fifteen million unchurched residents in public institutions, with people from every clime and of every color, don't we see here a most fruitful field ripe for harvest?

One may be trained correctly in a Christian home and church, learn to appreciate God's multiple blessings in life, willingly and faithfully attend the services of God's house, participate in the congregation's activities, and yet by uncontrollable circumstances become a scattered and wandering sheep.

Jake was such a one. A good Christian for many years, with a simple and deeply-rooted dedication to the Lord, even during his military service and long absence from home, he arrived at that stage in life when the weaknesses of age make one dependent upon others for daily necessities and niceties. All of Jake's relatives had died. His old friends were long gone. He was all alone in this big and menacing world. That can frighten even the most self-sufficient individual.

Reluctantly he applied for veterans' benefits, remembering the regimentation of army life with its cold and crisp effects. His application was accepted and processed, and soon Jake was a resident in a facility far removed from his former homestead. It wasn't really too difficult to adjust once again to domiciliary living with hundreds of other veterans. After all, he had shelter, clothing and food, and the minimal basics of existence. He had companionship, such as it was, and there was a lot of mechanical and impersonal entertainment offered to help pass the time. Yet, what do all these things truly mean as we watch for the shadows of the dark valley we all must walk through one day?

There were opportunities for worship on Sundays. Once or twice Jake went, because his soul was hungry and thirsty. But this wasn't the food he had been accustomed to. It was a "religion different from what I learned in my years in parochial school." Oh, yes, he read daily in his Bible and wore out his prayer books, but he felt like a sheep lost in the desert, far from the Shepherd's fold.

One day I met this stooped, handicapped man in one of the corridors at the Veterans' Hospital and Home and struck up a conversation with him. He was skeptical at first, but quickly warmed to our contact when he sensed that we were of a kindred spirit in speaking about future hopes. How happy he was to know that a pastor was available to help him fill the spiritual void in his life! As we discussed God's claim on our life, as we talked about the Savior's embracing love, we soon found that we were brothers in faith. Week by week that conviction grew, and as I introduced Jake to other men on the ward who confessed the same faith as we did, he soon became a communicant with our small group on that floor.

Go where you will, you will scarcely find a more serious and devoted listener to the call of the Good Shepherd. Life is ebbing out for this man, but there is that gleam of hope in his tired eyes. There will be a better tomorrow, not promised or fashioned by man but by a kind heavenly Father who restored all the blessings of paradise through his Son. Jake knows that he doesn't deserve this. He will tell you so. And maybe that's why he bows his head so low as from the innermost depths of his being. He repeats word for word the confession of sins at our monthly sacramental service. And how he delights in speaking the Creed, the Lord's Prayer, and the Benediction! All these have become much more than words to him. They are his life!

SEVENTY TIMES SEVEN

Little Henry grew up in a normal way in a good Christian home. His parents accepted him as a gift from God and saw to it that he, and the rest of the children in the family, received the best training in religion that they were able to provide with the help of the church. He was in God's house regularly; was baptized there; attended its day school; and was confirmed in his faith. He also graduated from a Lutheran high school, as did his brothers.

He was an industrious and ambitious young man, who had no problem in finding gainful employment. When he felt able, he took on the responsibilities of marriage and was wed to one of his schoolmates. It was a happy union and excellent companionship. Being serious-minded young people, the two built their castles in the air and looked forward to a long and profitable life, blessed by God.

They fared well for a number of years until a serious glandular disease ran uncontrollably through Hank's body. That is when the nasty problems began. He became grotesque in stature, very irritable in his discomforts, and very sullen as his coworkers and employers first made fun of him and later humiliated and abused him. The physical problems became increasingly severe, and Hank found it impossible to obtain employment paying enough to support his wife and family. The dutiful helpmeet and mother tried her best to help along, but bad went to worst, and there seemed no way out of the dilemma. The situation became critical when Hank, thoroughly broken in spirit, began begging for drinks at the corner tavern. At home he was unkempt, lazy, vile in speech, and abusive.

What do you do under conditions like this? The wife and children separated from Hank and went their own way. He continued to deteriorate. "Out of a sense of duty" he began to pilfer foodstuffs from stores. At the moment it seemed to be an allowable and easy way to survive. But the cancer of sin has its own way of growing secretly, and grow it did indeed in Hank. It wasn't long before he was in serious trouble with the law. He was sent to prison.

To him this was not legitimate punishment, which could result in a rediscovery of himself; it was merely relief from exceptional burdens he no longer cared to carry. Prison became a haven of physical rest. In fact, it became a way of life. You serve your time, are released into a hostile world, survive by committing another crime, and return to prison for rest. That was the pattern. Prison records, I believe, will show that Hank was incarcerated for a variety of offenses more than seventy times! This was life to Hank. What else was there for him?

Through the years this onetime child of God, sheep of the Shepherd's fold, had completely stopped his ears to the Shepherd's voice. Occasional pangs of conscience were quickly smothered as he tried to rationalize his "undeserved" lot. Not even the concentrated efforts of prison personnel to help right this man were of any avail. Stubbornly he charted his own course and was disliked and hated by most everyone.

How low can a man fall? How deep? During one of his releases, a deputy warden met Hank on the street of a nearby city and was asked for fifty cents "to tide me over." He was refused. A few minutes later there was a sound of shattering glass a short distance away. The warden walked to the spot and found Hank standing before a store window with a brick in his hand. He patiently waited for the police to arrest him and send him back to prison as a habitual offender! That would at least assure warm quarters for the winter months!

Then came the day when he was stricken with a severe heart attack and was rushed to the prison hospital in critical condition. There were good reasons to fear that he would not survive. The warden had his secretary pull Hank's file, and there he read that the man was of Lutheran "persuasion." This happened on a day when I was at the institution on my regular schedule. The secretary was watching, and when I entered the lobby she informed me of the situation.

Immediately I went to his hospital cell, told him who I was and what my purpose was in visiting. For the next ten minutes all I could do was listen to some of the vilest cursing I have ever heard. The dying man was so filled with hatred toward God and society that his lips could scarcely spit out all the venom. I wondered. I prayed for words from heaven. Then, very suddenly, Hank stopped speaking, but the curses seemed to keep bouncing back and forth in the small cell.

Words came to my lips from the heart. I could feel for this man and more so when in gasps he tried to tell me his life story. This was not a new experience—and thank God that it wasn't—else I might have failed miserably in trying to help this soul. He told me that his family had deserted him in his day of trouble; his parents were dead; his brothers refused to recognize him as being of their flesh and blood. He was alone, yes ALL alone!

It was easy to speak now about the One who had not forgotten, the Good Shepherd Jesus—that he was calling to Hank even now and offering his saving help. I told him about the limitless love of Jesus, which gives man the power to overcome the sad and crushing consequences of sin and guilt. I reminded him of man's many transgressions against a holy God and of our utter depravity and condemnation. Most of all, I tried to reassure him that still in this late hour of life the Savior was offering him pardon for every sin and the promise of heaven.

The man began to sob, and then cry loudly as a baby. Tears literally gushed from his pinched eyes. They were hot tears from hell poured through his lids by conscience. They were tears of shame as he remembered his God-forgetting activities. They were tears of humble repentance rifling down the hardened creases in his face. Best of all, they were tears of gratitude that come only when one is able to value the immensity of an undeserved gift. In Jesus' holy blood all of man's wretchedness and guilt is drowned, never again to rise up and damn him!

One could see that his strength was seeping away. Would it be minutes, or hours, or days before this sheep would be carried home? No one knew for sure. What we did know was that only the Word of the living God was the medicine needed in this critical hour. So we read it, especially as it applies to such a tender moment. The sobbing stopped. There was a somber silence in the prison cell, and only the prayers we prayed for him could be heard.

With great difficulty Hank turned his eyes toward me and whispered, "The Lord's Supper. May I?" Quickly we prepared the bedside table and the Communion elements. "This is my body given for you. This is my blood shed for you for the forgiveness of all your sins." And you could read peace in that troubled face. Believe me; I left that clanging door with a song in my heart! Our Good Shepherd had found another of the "other sheep" and would gently carry it home to the flock.

During that night the man died, as they told me, without a struggle. He slept away in the Shepherd's arms. There remained only the burial of the shell. And that posed another problem. Where? By whom? When the warden called early that morning he asked that I contact the brothers to make arrangements. He gave me their names and addresses. It took several hours to make the contacts, but not a one of them was concerned, nor would they accept any duty toward their brother. Mostly it was cold and stony silence.

Hank lies buried in a small plot provided by the state for unwanted people. He lies amid the trees of an apple orchard on state property, awaiting that great and glorious day of the resurrection, when all time is over on earth. Meanwhile his soul is singing the praises of the Shepherd, joining the angel choirs in the crescendo of the "Magnificat."

A STRANGER IN PARADISE

Freddi was almost twenty years old before he met the Good Shepherd. He had been following other shepherds who taught him many things that did him no good.

He was born of an illegitimate union in Germany, in the days of Adolph Hitler, and was thoroughly trained in the ideals of godless Nazism. He became a willing ward of the state and developed into an expert "goose-stepper" in the ranks of the infamous Jugendbund. The state was his family, especially after his mother deserted him and returned to her homeland in the U.S.A.

Nazism, of course, knew nothing about God or the Bible. It wrote its own code of morals in which it exalted the goals of German supremacy over the rest of the world. Actually, Hitler was the idol-god; everything he proclaimed was believed as truth. To us in America, this is unthinkable and unbelievable. But given the proper climate in politics and economics, the seeds of dictatorship will grow to dominate and enslave a whole society.

Freddi grew up as a noxious weed thriving in the atmosphere of hate and warfare. He had never heard God say: "Thou shall have no other gods." He had no god but Hitler. He knew no sin but transgression of the Fuehrer's wishes and orders. So he needed no savior beyond the good graces of the Bund to which he had pledged absolute loyalty. We might say that he had a shepherd of sorts, but one who couldn't lead him to the "green pastures and still waters." Rather, he was being led to the scorched earth and dried rivers of dedicated fanaticism and the shedding of other sheep's blood. THE STATE IS GOD! At all costs the warped ideals of the Hitlerian Vaterland must prevail. That's the air this youth breathed in his strange shepherd's fold.

Shortly before World War II broke out, his mother in America had pangs of conscience about deserting her son. As the war clouds blackened she returned to Germany, located the youth after some searching, and somehow managed to get permission to bring him back with her to her home in America. It seems that her citizenship covered also her son, now almost eighteen years old. And suddenly, protesting Freddi was no longer a Nazi, but a member of a nation he had been taught to hate with a passion! What a traumatic experience for the lad.

Our nation at that time was drafting its young people into the armed services and training them for combat duty. Legally, Freddi was eligible for inclusion in the draft, and when his number was drawn, he was called for training. Imagine his consternation! He had many fears and was awed by his duty to our government. Reluctantly, he swore allegiance to the United States and promised to defend it against all enemies.

His life became a nightmare in the training camps. He did not understand the English language well and consequently failed miserably in many assignments. Because of his unmistakable German accent, his fellow-trainees made him the butt of much horseplay; many jibes were directed at him; tricks (and some were not at all innocent fun) were played on him; and he suffered much maltreatment. He soon hated the government, the American system, and he hated his mother and himself for being where he was.

It was not at all unusual, that under such pressures of body and mind, Freddi's health broke down. His body was weak, his spirit shattered, and before long he was hospitalized with a severe case of malnutrition and general debility. A few weeks later his condition was diagnosed as tuberculosis, and he was placed into an isolation ward. According to military medical services he was transferred from one hospital to another, all in strange cities. No wonder that he was lonely (for reasons of her own, his mother was out of contact), fearful and sullen, irritable, and then withdrawn to the point of not communicating at all with those compassionate people who were trying their utmost to help him fight his battles for health.

I met this "other sheep" at Wood Veterans' Hospital at a time when his condition had become critical. The tuberculosis was far advanced and defied any treatment known at that time.

The case was terminal, and Freddi lost whatever little hope he might have had.

One afternoon a nurse, who was trying so hard to gain his confidence, but with no success, asked me to see Freddi. She knew that I could speak his native tongue and thought this might be a breakthrough to all misery locked up in her patient's body and mind. Gladly I responded and called on the youth. And never, never, from thousands of patients I was privileged to visit, did I ever receive an icier reception! Even when I spoke German he kept his face toward the wall, except for an occasional furtive glance. It was as though he was sizing me up, not knowing what to expect from one who came to talk about God. Would I talk about Hitler? about our president? Who is God, and what does he want in my life? Such, no doubt, were the thoughts that added to Freddi's confusion and fears.

Right from the very start, I wanted him to know my purpose in calling, and so I spoke very simply about our God, our alienation from him through sin, our well-deserved punishment and condemnation in life and in death. But I never left his room without telling him of God's great love, his forgiveness through Christ Jesus, and our gift of freedom from the power of every enemy of man's soul. Yet, after each of my many visits, I sensed his indifference. Perhaps he didn't listen at all during those first short calls. Surely there was no evidence of any positive response.

What it was that brought the turning point I do not know. Maybe it was my asking his permission to speak my prayers for him in his hearing. Maybe it was a growing trust in my desire to be of help. And yet, I do know what made his attitude change. It was the Word being used by the Holy Spirit to melt the iciness in his twisted mind and stony heart. After several weeks you could see the seed sending out tender sprouts. Barriers were breaking down, and at times he would speak a few words. Sometimes they were comments, sometimes questions, but at last the lines of communication were opening up. He was beginning to trust.

Then one day I threatened to stop wasting his and my time in his room. It was only a ploy on my part, but he completely surprised me by releasing a torrent of hidden feelings and emotions. He was afraid! He was afraid of himself, of his "enemy" doctors and nurses and social workers, afraid of me and of God whom I represented. His words became a tearful plea for help to remove the tons of crushing afflictions that rested on him. From then on it was a pleasure and an undeserved privilege to call on him. He was like a dry sponge capable of soaking up much water. He was eager to hear the Scriptures tell him that he was a redeemed child of the one true God. He beamed at the stories of the Good Shepherd's love and loyalty. The story of the cross enchanted him. The gospel was for him! "Come unto me."

Together we read many portions of the Bible in German and in English. We studied the Catechism with its simple questions and answers. We read many hymn verses, some of which he memorized and repeated during long sleepless nights. We prayed many prayers in which we asked for God's help and guidance. I waited patiently, and finally it came: "Can I be baptized?" Oh, what a happy day! Sincere and deep was the confession of faith in his Shepherd-God when Freddi promised to follow him through the valley of the shadow of death.

By faith a Nazi God-hater was now a saint in the family of God—all through the power of the means of grace. "The power of God unto salvation" was the way St. Paul put it. It is the only power that can save us from eternal death.

There was no renewal of physical strength for Freddi, but his soul was reborn and healthy, strong to face the fact of inevitable death and judgment. At his request I bought him two small candlesticks and candles, a wooden cross, a new bilingual Catechism, a hymnbook, and a Bible. All these he proudly displayed on his small bedside table as a mighty testimony to all who entered his room. He was a CHRISTIAN. His few remaining weeks became a lesson for all.

The disease progressed rather rapidly and soon carried its victim to the grave. Freddi was buried with Christian rites by one of our pastors far away in another state. Our letters to his mother and to her pastor brought responses of much gratitude. The mother was ashamed, but repentant. Her pastor felt the joy of being assured that another sinner had repented and found his Lord. Most important to all of us was the fact that a lost sheep had by grace found the peace which passes all human under-standing. For Freddi it was peace brought to an unusually trou-bled and tried soul by the Good Shepherd.

IT CAN HAPPEN TO ALL

Carla's roots were in a good family of professing and prac-ticing Christians. She was well-trained in the fundamentals of God's truth. As a result she was a complete person who enjoyed her daily activities, casting all her cares on a faithful Helper, her Shepherd Jesus.

But the gradual and then swifter passing of the years has a way of deceiving us and keeping us from much serious contem-plation. How and where will we live one day when we are alone in the world and our family and close friends have passed from the earthly scene? Carla, in her trusting and carefree spirit, was a victim of careless planning, or little planning at all.

In her old age she realized that she had a few dollars, but no home; no place to stay; no friends "to talk things out with;" no relatives who might provide advice and companionship. Fortu-nately, through public welfare agencies arrangements were made to house her and provide for her in a large public residential cen-ter. It was shelter, food, clothing and care, but nothing nearly like the places she formerly called "home."

Worst of all, she complained, was the fact that she was many miles from her church, and there was just no way for her to get there. This was a major disappointment for her. Oh, yes, her pastor called on occasion, comforted her and served her Communion. But, and this happens far too often, for a variety of reasons she was transferred from one home to another, and in her forgetful-ness she did not always let the pastor know her new address.

The faithful pastor accepted a call and moved to another city, and his successor did not feel the same responsibility toward Carla to continue to search for this wandering sheep from move to move. She became a lost sheep! It was not that she easily for-got her Lord, but her sense of belonging to God's family was dulled almost to the point of extinction. Her strength was failing, her memory no longer alert or reliable, and she began to live in a spiritual limbo.

Once again she was transferred, this time to a new, large and comfortable place. By this time it really didn't matter much to her where or how she lived. For her the sand in the hourglass was running low. But, on one of her first days at this home, she heard an announcement over the audio system that Lutheran services would be held that afternoon in the chapel area. Could it be that this might fill the void in her life? She was curious enough to attend the services, and she once again heard the voice of her Good Shepherd! She recognized it well—in the liturgy, the hymns, the prayers, and the sermon. HE is here!

After the service was over, I met Carla and heard her tale of woe and want. It brought tears to my eyes to hear again how the realities and cruelties of our earthly existence can shrivel, even kill, an immortal soul. What a challenge to the shepherds of our day to leave, if necessary, the "ninety and nine in the wilderness and search for the one sheep that is lost."

Many visits with Carla followed. The emptied heart needed to be refilled with the bread and water of life. The color of spiritual health became more and more evident as she realized, happily, that though she had been forgotten by many, her Good Shepherd had never let her slip out of his sight. In him she found her secure hiding place, safe from Satan's attempts to destroy her soul.

Today, Carla is in attendance at every service we provide at the home, and rarely is she absent from the regular Communion services. The body and blood of Jesus, given and shed for the remission of her sins, is a "must" for her as she walks at age eighty-eight down the path that becomes narrower and narrower.

One of the many fruits of her restored faith is the dime or quarter she reverently places on the altar after each worship service. The world may never become aware of her as a dignified and important individual, and that is not important either. God knows and looks with pleasure on her simple ways of glorifying his saving name.

RICHES TO RAGS TO RICHES

Psalm 119:67, 71 states, "Before I was afflicted I went astray, but now I obey your word . . . . It was good for me to be afflicted so that I might learn your decrees." Many contented Christians would subscribe wholeheartedly to the truth of these inspired words. Jack would be one of them.

He was a sheep born into the flock through staunch, dedicated parental believers and supporters of the church and its work. Every opportunity to get to know the Good Shepherd was set before him lovingly, and he happily accepted them all. He was the kind of child who deeply respected his parents and without complaint followed their directions. Christian day school and Sunday school were a delight for him. And after he graduated from Lutheran high school he spent most of his leisure time at church attending meetings of the youth group and promoting programs of Christian fellowship. He felt at home in this atmosphere and was content and happy in the sheepfold.

In later years those memories were a real asset in his attempt to recapture the sense of spiritual security he once had. One of the special remembrances of childhood days was the trip, a very long streetcar ride from one end of the city to the other, which his mother insisted on making each Sunday afternoon to the Poor Farm in Wauwatosa. He and his sister went along to help carry the wicker basket filled with goodies—Kaffekuchen and cookies and fruits. These they would share with some of the aged residents who had no other friends or visitors. When they returned home late Sunday afternoon the whole family had that warm and satisfying feeling that comes with services rendered to the less fortunate.

But things change. After father and mother died, there was a feeling of irreplaceable loss and disappointment at the break in the family circle. Jack especially felt a growing anger at what God had permitted to happen. In his resentment, he turned to other activities apart from the church and its good steadying influences. His contacts with brothers and sisters became fewer and fewer. He was on his own, carving out his niche in life.

When he entered the business world to make his living, married a celebrity (a Ziegfeld Girl, for the benefit of our older readers) and fathered a beautiful daughter, all the old and good influences were replaced by new ones that led him down the slippery road of materialism. The driving forces of "What shall we eat and drink; how can I earn more to support our lifestyle; what new pleasures can we enjoy?" took precedence. He soon forgot that true riches are always rooted in God and his gifts to men, particularly the gift of all gifts: the Good Shepherd Jesus. Forgetting this is one of the strong tools Satan employs to destroy souls. An oversupply of this world's goods can be a real dangerous enemy.

Suddenly, a startling thing happened. Jack's employer died, and when the will was probated, Jack became sole owner of the business and, in addition, was bequeathed the sum of $50,000 in cash and securities. Probably, that is not much in our day's inflated economy, but at the time it was a priceless treasure for one who had never managed to save much. Besides, the business was growing by leaps and bounds, profits were multiplying, and Jack became a moderately wealthy man.

In the whirl of worldliness that followed, Jack developed some very bad habits. He began to drink and gamble daily. He neglected his business, lost his reliable employees, and was estranged from his wife and daughter.

I met Jack one morning after a chapel service at General Hospital. He looked so sick and so sad that it must have been quite an effort for him to attend. After the service, he waited for the others to leave and then asked for a few minutes of "serious talk." Believe me, we did talk—and seriously, not only that morning, but for hours during the weeks of his stay at the hospital. I listened through the whole tragic story and could hear this lost sheep crying out for relief from its agony of separation from the Shepherd. He was a charity patient at the Hospital, broken down in health with infections and diseases brought on mainly by his careless dissipations. He was an emotional wreck since his wife and daughter had left him, and in financial ruin after the business had fallen apart and the $50,000 was gone. He was also facing spiritual death because he had sinned so terribly against conscience and truth. The once mighty man was a poor beggar now, without enough money to buy a bottle of aspirin to fight his pain!

"I don't know what moved me to attend church that morning," he told me, "but I'm happy that I did. You preached a sermon I wish I could have heard many times over. You spoke about riches that moth and rust can corrupt and destroy, and then you told us about indestructible riches that nothing can spoil, and you urged us to seek and find and lay up treasures in heaven. I felt you were speaking directly to me; rather, God was appealing in love and unlimited mercy. Will you please help me get back on the right road? I am so sorry that I threw away my anchor of God's Word and lost myself in earthly pleasures. When I should have been thanking him for all my blessings, I forgot him and trusted in my own brand of security. How can we remake my life, if that is possible at this late date? As God gives me pardon and strength, I want to return to my church; I want to be with my family again and be useful to them. I want to have my sixteen-year-old daughter instructed and confirmed, and lead my wife, who is of another faith, into the family of God."

All this and more had come into his mind as he listened intently to God's Word that Sunday. And I shudder to think of what might have happened or not happened if we had not had the privilege of conducting services at that hospital, and just at that time! A lost sheep would have been searching and listening, but would not have heard the Shepherd's voice.

Jack became a different man. Day by day he was recapturing those truths once so familiar to him. In his affliction, God brought him back through the eternal Word to paths of right living and peace. God used an undershepherd to help him reestablish himself and overcome the shame and disgrace of the past. As he recovered from his illness, he again found employment, began to support his family, and kept his promise to have his daughter instructed in the ways of the Lord. In fact, he attended all classes with her and experienced the happy day of her confirmation.

He died a few years later. What a happy homecoming it must have been! His one disappointment was that he had not been able to convince his wife to hear the Shepherd's voice. This she told me years later, when she called one day from her room in a shabby hotel, in which she was living out her last days. She had never been able to shake off the tinsel and glitter of her former life as a wined and dined popular performer. Worldly idealism had fastened its straps about her, and she never could understand "religion." Yet, wasn't her unexpected phone calling really a cry of sorts for help to find peace and hope for the life to come?

We worked with her for some time, speaking the truth in love, praying that the Shepherd might somehow rescue this perishing soul. She disappeared, and we never again heard from or of her. Our consolation is that the good seed was sown. We hope that it sprouted and grew, but we shall never know for sure this side of heaven.

How humbly, how fervently we ought to use the prayer-hymn:

> *In the hour of trial, Jesus, plead for me*
> *Lest by base denial I unworthy be.*
> *When you see me waver, with a look recall,*
> *Nor for fear or favor ever let me fall*
>
> *With forbidden pleasures should this vain world charm*
> *Or its tempting treasures Spread to work me harm,*
> *Bring to my remembrance Sad Gethsemane*
> *Or, in darker semblance, Cross-crowned Calvary.*
>
> *Should your mercy send me Sorrow, toil, and woe,*
> *Or should pain attend me on my path below,*
> *Grant that I may never fail your cross to view;*
> *Grant that I may ever cast my care on you.*
>
> *When my life is ending, though in grief or pain,*
> *When my body changes Back to dust again,*
> *On your truth relying, through that mortal strife,*
> *Jesus, take me, dying, to eternal life.*

PHYSICALLY ILL SHEEP

Very few of us remain strangers to physical illnesses, diseases, or accidents. Since Eden, and its unforgettable happenings, even a famous child of God like Job must feel the sting of pains and distresses. (Read his story in the Old Testament book of Job for details.)

Christians understand that God permits and uses our physical troubles in his own merciful way, both as chastisements and as means to cultivate a firmer faith in his salvation. He also uses them to bring disguised blessings. Sometimes the ills are minimal, and a quick recovery follows. At other times they are severe and terminal, defying all medical science. Every good shepherd, who is alert to the total needs of his flock, will recognize symptoms that demand his special attention, lest they turn into crises and chronic disability. With whatever means at his disposal, the shepherd tends his sheep and seeks to ease the disease. Christian faith recognizes that sicknesses are sent from God; Christian love uses them as opportunities for kindness and compassion.

EVEN TO HOAR HAIRS

For many years, Norma had been blessed with a healthy and happy life. Her family was her pride and joy. Her church stood at the center of her thinking and doing. Without any previous warnings, there came the awful day when she suddenly collapsed and was rushed to the hospital. Stroke!

All the kindly care of the professionals and the steady ministrations of her pastor helped immensely, but they could not remove the residual paralysis and the incapacitation that accompanied it. At first, it was not too great a burden. Faith was mighty, and understanding friends and family helped to carry the cross.

But when the malady lingered through months and years, Norma received less and less attention. Finally she had to battle her problem alone.

First there was a convalescent home; later a nursing home. At age eighty with family gone and friends dead, the lamp of life flickered low. Norma was placed into the strange surroundings of a Catholic residence for the aged.

She lived there for more than a year before her case came to our attention. A former neighbor accidentally located her, called on her, and then asked a pastor to visit her. The pastor referred the case to me.

What joys elated that shriveling soul, as lonely Norma realized that her Shepherd had sought her out to refresh her parched spirit! How eager she was to hear Scripture readings, hymns, and prayers! And the crown of it all was to again receive the body and blood of her Lord in the sacrament after years of isolation.

Today, Norma sits in her small room as most of life passes her by. Yet she confidently awaits the day when her difficult earthly journey will be over and she can close her eyes in peaceful death.

On a regular schedule, she is visited and communed. Though very limited in sight and hearing, she sees the star that led the Magi to Christ's cradle, and she hears the angels' song: "Glory to God in the highest, and on earth peace." Her drawn lips still manage a smile when she is told: "Your pastor has come to see you."

Remember in your prayers the thousands of Norma's in the world!

EDUCATION AT THE BRINK OF ETERNITY

Dick was a young man, twenty-seven years of age and married, and a student at a state university. In boyhood days he had gone through all the formal steps of Christian education, and for several years was very active in church life. In his good family surroundings, he was sure to be a sheep that would graze healthily in the Shepherd's pastures.

But strange things can happen in a relatively short period of time. They did happen in Dick's case. He was not at all suspicious, nor particularly watchful, on the path of higher education, which promised to lead him to a profitable professional career. He gave no thought to devilish devices set to trap him. He wasn't skeptical of the confusions created and nurtured in a bright young mind being trained in an agnostic and atheistic educational system. Almost without realizing that something was happening to him, Dick fell into a web that might have destroyed his soul.

At first, he would question some of the anti-God statements of his professor; sometimes openly disagree with them. But, bit by bit, the seeds of unbelief and the exaltation of human reason grew into producing plants. His questions and objections became silent before the mighty pressures of "higher wisdom" and the mind-conceit of his peers, who seemed wiser than the simplistic truths of God, as taught in the Bible. In short order Dick was outside the fold.

But the Shepherd was watching! After a brilliant start in his classes, with scholastic honors heaped upon him and with visions of great success for the future, the Shepherd moved into action in Dick's life and began his work of spiritual restoration.

Dick became ill. It was nothing serious at first, just a worn body and an exhausted mind. Rest and treatment would put him back on track soon. But, day by day and week by week, there was no progress in the fight for health and the prognosis was not optimistic at all. Instead, it indicated a steady and deadly deterioration. Dick's doctor hospitalized him for complete tests and intensive observation. And after about a week the diagnosis was settled on by the staff of the hospital. It had to be shocking to a young man ready to conquer the world with know-how and zeal. "CANCER!" the report said. The disease had already ravaged vital organs and was spreading very fast. The experts predicted only a few more months of life for Dick.

Bitterness and resentment flowed from his lips and out of his shattered heart. He became noncooperative and abusive. Even the nurses were reluctant to enter his room because of his rantings and ravings. His young wife and other relatives often left the room in tears.

One evening, an understanding Christian nurse called my attention to this problem patient and asked that I see him. I was willing, but after the first visit I must admit that it would have been easy to pass by his door without looking in. He was angry and fighting the world of science, whose god of self-interest and self-sufficiency had collapsed at Dick's feet. And then, probably with deeper resentment, he was fighting God himself with the charge of injustice.

It was not easy, but it was surely necessary to try to help this young man out of his hopeless wilderness. Praying for understanding, patience, strength, and tactful wisdom, I called on the young man for many days and pointed him to the basic truths of God's Word, as they help us understand ourselves and God in his dealings with us undeserving sinners. In this case, the Lord's promise that his Word shall never return unto him void came alive before our eyes. Gradually, the fighting and abuse diminished and then stopped entirely, as Dick reabsorbed the import of the Word he had been taught long ago.

God owes us nothing. We are rebels, transgressors of his holy will and ways. We owe him everything, but we cannot ever pay our debt. His justice must condemn us in life and in death. Yet, God made it possible to neutralize and even reverse the effects of our condemnation, by having his Son Jesus pay the awful price on Calvary. Now if we believe this, trust his promises, follow him, consign our life to him, he will use all things that happen to us in life for our good, never for evil. He will not, he cannot again exact payment for a debt that has been paid for us. Even death in youth is good and blessed in God's higher wisdom, applied to us as we follow the Lamb that was slain for us.

Dick understood this through the working of the Holy Spirit, and in the remaining few weeks of his earthly pilgrimage, he prepared himself diligently for death by filling up the well of faith with the water of life; the assurances of a truthful and gracious Father in heaven.

Since he had previously willed his body to a medical school for research, the family had to content itself with a memorial service in one of our churches. But it was a glorious service, glorifying God and his Word, the Word that turns hearts and souls to a longsuffering and gentle Shepherd's love and care.

MERCY FOR A TROUBLED LIFE

This side of heaven no one will ever know perfection, no, not even a Christian. And circumstances in life may so warp his judgment that he is able to choose wrong paths, forgetting to ask himself always: "What would my Lord direct me to do in my present problem?" Not remembering that simple question can lead to much heartache and a rocky pilgrimage through our average "three score and ten."

This story is about Peter, a happily married man, the father of several children, an active churchman. He was not the executive type, not overly ambitious for more and more of this world's goods, but faithful and industrious in the job that supported the happy family. He was grateful to God for all his blessings of body and soul, and expressed his thanks by making Sunday morning the chief event of each week. He and his family thanked the Lord for the privilege of hearing the Shepherd's voice and being reassured that they were indeed the children of God. The family prayed together, worshiped together, stayed together, and served the Lord together at every opportunity.

Deep troubles and multiple problems surfaced, however, when the wife and mother of the family was stricken with a variety of maladies, became a chronic invalid in middle age, and then died within a year. The blow was a heavy one, and it almost crushed Peter, especially when the problems of raising the young ones became his solid responsibility. The challenge was not easy, and Peter never really was able to cope with it.

A day of heartbreak it was, when the children had to be placed into a care home. There was many a tearful farewell on the weekends, when father went to visit the children. Added to this was the financial need to pay for their care. No wonder that he developed lasting furrows in his brow! As the tensions increased and the loneliness was overpowering, he felt totally drained and deserted, and it was no longer a simple thing to pray for guidance and vigor.

While waiting his turn in a barber shop one day, he paged through magazines that carried ads inviting single men and women to join lonely hearts clubs, and by the pen-pal method, possibly find a marriage partner. His thoughts turned to the numbers of people who were as lonely as he. The thoughts were intriguing to the point that he copied the address of one of the clubs and later that night wrote a letter applying for membership. Years later he wished he had never opened that magazine.

Letter after letter soon arrived, mainly from women in the eastern part of the country, offering themselves as marriage partners, sight unseen, and making enticing promises. One letter, of the many, seemed to suit his circumstances very well. He answered it, and that led to longer correspondence and an eventual meeting in person. The woman appeared to be so sincere and so Christian in spirit, that Peter proposed marriage in the hope that he might recapture at least a part of his former happy family life. And the marriage was a success—but for only two years. By that time the new wife had become tired of mothering Peter's children.

There was much bitter bickering and argument until, finally, the wife and substitute mother left Peter's home. The note on the kitchen table said: "I am tired and disappointed. Please do not try to find me; I'm going away for good." Peter was utterly frustrated, angry, and his mind filled with thoughts of revenge. He struck out against the world, against God, and against women in particular by committing the horrible sin of violating his oldest daughter!

After his trial in court, the judge sentenced him to the maximum penalty for the offense, twenty-five years in prison, and years of increasing degradation for this once fine Christian man. He just fell apart physically, mentally, and spiritually. And then the great Good Shepherd reached out to his erring sheep.

I took particular note of him at the first chapel service he attended in prison. He struck my eye as one who shouldn't be there; he was not at all the usual type of offender. In an interview that day, he told me his sordid story of weakness and shame. As he talked, it was as though a ton of care was being lifted from his shoulders. Out of his heavy heart came the tears of remorse and sorrow for his sin. How could he have forgotten his God so completely? My stomach churned, and I became nauseated at the revelation of his inexcusable guilt. But you must forget self when dealing with a sheep precious to the Master. So I proceeded, as in so many other cases at other times, to speak of sin and grace, pleading prayer and pardon at the hands of One who can forgive and who hides our offenses in the depths of the sea. Peter's humble confession was followed by a reborn faith and hope. He would see this through, grateful for the Shepherd's help. It was a pleasure to work with this man in the years that followed, if one can speak of pleasure in connection with the steady sight of human depravity, such as is shown behind prison walls. But we were happy after every visit. Peter's case strengthened us in our ministry and gave us new incentives to carry on in a work that often left us exhausted in an attempt to deal, evangelically, with people whose sins you had to hate with a passion. Yet when dealing with such transgressions, we must humbly admit, "There but for the grace of God go I."

Satan had tested and sifted this man, but God prevailed! And the subsequent happenings in Peter's life were further evidences of the Lord's work in him. He wrote regularly to his children and was thrilled at the rare visits allowed with them on special days. He became concerned too about the spiritual welfare of the wife who had walked out on him. He was anxious to forgive her, even as he had been forgiven so richly, though he realized that perhaps never would he be reunited with her.

The wife had disappeared, as she had threatened in her note to Peter the day she left his home. But nobody is able to hide from the Good Shepherd, as we learned quite unexpectedly one morning when I noticed her name on the list of new admissions to a local specialty hospital. The name was the same, but could it really be Peter's wife? I went to her room, established the relationship connections, and after a time was able, under God, to lead her back to her Shepherd. Her restoration meant relief for a troubled conscience and the easing of a sense of great guilt. Another lost sheep found and led into the fold!

Through a bit of honest manipulation, we were instruments in bringing Peter and his wife together in the presence of the family. It was a sensitive visit that ended happily, with all pledging new loyalty to the Shepherd.

Then, after a short walk on a straight road, Peter suffered another devastating shock. His reconciled wife died very suddenly. It was all too much. The pressures deranged his mind. On release from prison, he found temporary lodging in a cheap "flea-bag" hotel, but soon was adjudged a chronic mental health case and was confined to an asylum, where he lived out his years in fright and terrible delusions. Now and then there was a lucid period during which the Word of the Shepherd penetrated the barriers in his mind. And, at long last, the Good Shepherd called a halt to all ills and carried his bruised and wounded sheep home. It was an unusual burial service, a happy one! The children and I couldn't but thank and praise God for his many mercies in the midst of a messy life; Peter was at rest! "Ashes to ashes, dust to dust," in the firm hope that the better days will come when body and soul, reunited, will live in the complete and perfect home in heaven.

VETERANS OF OUR WARS

As good citizens of our country, we want to show our appreciation to the men and women who have fought our wars for us. In many respects, we treat them royally and grant them special privileges for their services. One valuable thing we offer them is the care available in a whole network of government hospitals and homes maintained for them in their days of illness or disability.

As a church, dare we forget that man does not live by bread alone? He lives the abundant life, only when every word from the mouth of a gracious God is brought to him—the call of the Good Shepherd, if you will. Then not just this life is enriched for him but also the perfect life beyond the grave may be his inheritance.

One of our institutions was known years ago as the old "Soldiers' Home." Much more modern hospital facilities have been built there in recent years for the care of veterans. And the national cemetery on the grounds is available for burial to any who has served his or her country in time of war. Some veterans make the rebuilt Domiciliary Barracks their permanent home in their later years.

I remember the compound well from boyhood days. As a special treat, on a sunny summer Sunday afternoon, my parents would take us to the band concerts held out in the open for the entertainment of exsoldiers and the public. Little did I realize then that the blackening brick walls of the ornate old buildings housed and hid thousands of men who had earned care and keep by their military service. They had no other home. This was the end of the road for many.

In 1938 I was introduced to the real needs of these residents, when I was assigned to serve there as a Lutheran pastor. To this day, my heart goes out to the hidden-away souls living out their days there in comparative solitude. Quite a few are from surrounding states, far removed from the scenes of their childhood. Many try to keep busy remembering the past, just so that they might forget the present and future. Can we imagine the inner feelings of an aged and sick former colonel confined to a ward of many beds for chronic patients? Once honored and feted as a public servant, he is now "the patient in bed 40 next to the window." Or the man who once proudly rode his horse in the cavalry unit now being propelled to the dining area in a wheelchair? Or the man, who used to retire old army trucks with new hard rubber rims, now waits hopefully for a new pair of bedroom slippers? There they are, hundreds of men, young and old, from past wars, maimed, crippled, and many amputees! Some try to battle the boredom by draining the bottle; others turn to any available pain-easing drug.

Here too are sheep of the Shepherd's fold. They need spiritual food and drink. Although the government provides ample opportunities for participation in religious rites, men well-grounded in the knowledge of their Shepherd Jesus consistently remark that they do not hear his voice in multitudes of ecumenical observances. Is the fold so far away? Has the Shepherd forgotten?

Charley often asked himself that question. When he had become a chronic invalid his wife divorced him for "cruel and inhuman treatment," and his children too soon forgot about him "out there in the home far away." His bed was one of about thirty in an old-fashioned high-ceilinged room. The locker next to the bed contained all his earthly possessions, and the foot locker held his valuables.

A pastor from Chicago wrote saying that he had been told of this man and his Lutheran background, and would I please make contact. I did. And what I found was a gentle and loyal sheep, eager to graze in the pleasant pastures of the flock. He had problems, many of them and of various kinds. Admittedly, his greatest problem was sin and its fruits. And how do you still a conscience aroused by self-accusations? How do you avoid temptations that can be deadly? How do you restore hope?

The answers are there—in the Bible, God's Word, in pastoral counseling, and in the ministry of the sacrament. Charley has found a reason for continuing the battle of life. There's a glorious goal to be reached!

MEETING FOR WORSHIP

Today, strange little "congregations" gather in different units of the Veterans' Hospital for group meditations, or for the reception of Holy Communion. They may number from three to five members, all with one thing in common: They have the same Good Shepherd. The setting is usually a small dining room, and the churchly equipment is necessarily minimal. Sometimes a service with Communion may be held in the six by six foot "Poppy Room" of the Barracks, or even in the tiny mail room of an old building.

The attendees all have disabilities that confine them to wheelchairs or the use of crutches for their ambling around the ward. Each case is different, but the common denominator is faith in our Lord Jesus Christ who alone puts meaning into our existence. Occasionally, there may be an empty chair. One of the aged veterans has gone from the church militant to the church triumphant. Soon his place is occupied by a new admission to the ward, or by a new sheep that has been reclaimed by the Chief Shepherd. One by one, the lost are found at the direction of him who died for all.

The service is always impressive, made so by the openly shown sincerity of the worshipers. Most of everything we call life is in the past for them, but the future holds tremendous promise. Their sights are set on heaven. When Holy Communion is celebrated, most of the attendees join the pastor in the

54

Confession of Sins, they listen intently to the Absolution, and they speak the Creed and Lord's Prayer in unison. At the Benediction, they bow their heads low in reverent reception of the Savior's blessing.

And when the service is over, we feel like we have been in a great cathedral somewhere, drinking in the read and spoken Word, feeling all the while that we are part of a huge congregation telling our God how grateful we are for his love and care. We are!

FROM TRAGEDY TO TRIUMPH

Some claim to have power to foretell the future. Others wish they had such power. But, in his wisdom, the Lord does not unveil such knowledge to us. The suicide rate would climb unbelievably if it were possible for us to know everything that could and most likely will happen in years to come. How much wiser it is to live each day in the fear and trust of our Good Shepherd, who will lead us in all ways, good or bad, to his Father's mansions.

If young Art would have known the future course of his life, he would have been crushed in spirit to the point of ending his days very early in time. I say this in spite of the fact that he was of excellent character and deep Christian commitment, a reflection of the solid Christian home in which he grew up.

Soon after graduation, with honors, from high school, his talents were in demand in several career fields and the future held much promise. In his healthy enthusiasm, he looked ahead to a pleasant life under the continued blessings of his God. Little did he suspect that his road would have many unusual twists and turns, and little could he suspect, how hurting and cruel even a child of God's course could be.

Before all this happy and productive life could begin, Art was drafted into military service in World War II. On completion of his basic and advanced training, Art became an ace pilot in the Air Force and the leader of a bombing squad. He hated bombing; he hated bloodshed and killing; he hated war! But by his Lord's will expressed in Romans 13 (obedience to government), he was quietly submissive to his superior's orders and flew off to spread destruction and death on the enemy of our nation.

Many a young man in those days returned home a hero bedecked with ribbons and stripes and pins for outstanding and brave service. And many came back in a burial vault covered by the American flag. And many more came back maimed and crippled, without arms or legs, or with injuries that would take years to heal.

Art came home as one of these latter soldiers. His bomber had been riddled by the enemy's flak, hurtled to the ground in flames, and before being rescued, he and his crew suffered serious injuries and bad burns. Art was in critical condition and blind! For several months, he lay on hospital beds in different parts of the country, and then he was transferred to Wood Hospital in Milwaukee. There he received the newest in treatments for third-degree burns and also for a developing mental instability. Yet there seemed to be no progress at all, and so Art withdrew into a shell of isolation. He wouldn't converse with anyone, not even with his loving mother, who had taken up residence near the hospital so that she could visit him every day.

In my visits to his bedside, there seemed to be no recognition of what was being done or said by me or by his mother. But I never left his side without quoting pertinent passages of Scripture, which reminded son and mother of the Shepherd's promises, such as: "So do not fear, for I am with you; do not be dismayed, for I am your God. I will strengthen you and help you; I will uphold you with my righteous right hand" and "Do not fear, for I have redeemed you; I have summoned you by name; you are mine. When you pass through the waters, I will be with you; and when you pass through the rivers, they will not sweep over you. When you walk through the fire, you will not be burned; the flames will not set you ablaze" (Isaiah 41:10; 43:1, 2). And, of course, we always poured out our hearts in prayer.

This went on for months, seemingly without effect. Then, one afternoon, the mother called me and jubilantly told me that there were definite signs that Art's eyesight was returning. He had recognized her and had begun to speak single words. I hurried to his room and for the first time saw his unbandaged eyes; they almost appeared to be smiley eyes as they turned toward me. A tear or two were evident as we thanked God profusely.

With this encouragement, however, we were not ready for the awful developments of the next two weeks. During that time, as the eyesight improved miraculously, the condition of mind deteriorated very swiftly. There were times when Art was totally irrational and sometimes in a coma! Again we stood by, feeling our helplessness, but trusting the Shepherd who laid down his life for us. Though Art often ranted and raved, he became strangely quiet when he heard my voice speaking the things of God. "I lift up my eyes to the mountains—where does my help come from? My help comes from the Lord, the Maker of heaven and earth. He will not let your foot slip—he who watches over you will not slumber" (Psalm 121:1-3).

There were weeks on end of similar ministration, sometimes frequent, sometimes intermittent. It all seemed to be so hopeless! But then again one afternoon the mother called, and her words almost leaped over the wire: "Art has come out of his world of depression. It must be a miracle! Please stop in today." I did, and could scarcely believe what I saw and heard. The young man was trying hard to frame rational words and thoughts with his encrusted lips. And he made it! For the first time he could respond to direct questions and join us, with great effort, in speaking our Lord's Prayer and speaking his "amens" to other prayers of gratitude.

After that there was rapid progress, so rapid in fact that Art was allowed to transfer to a hospital in his home town upstate, where the encouragement of his family and many friends helped his convalescence and steady return to health.

Before leaving Milwaukee, Art called to ask if I could come to see him. I was glad to go. What he had to say was a lesson nobody should ever forget. In all his days of despondency his only hope was in the help of God, even though, too often, he could not express that in words. Life during those months was like a long black tunnel without a speck of light at either end. But quite often, in rational hours, a voice reverberated in the tunnel. I was the voice of God calling "Fear not! Fear not!" It was like the "valley of the shadow of death," and the strength to survive came from the Shepherd's "rod and staff" (Paraphrased from Psalm 23:4).

The Good Shepherd had led this life in a strange way, but he never forgot his precious sheep. "The Lord will keep you from all harm—he will watch over your life" (Psalm 121:7).

LEARNING THE FATHER'S BUSINESS

"The Lord disciplines the one he loves, and he chastens everyone he accepts as his son" (Hebrews 12:6).

We often wonder, don't we, why the Lord lets his hand fall so heavily on certain people? And how often do we hear it asked by the afflicted: "Why must this happen to me?" Only the Lord knows the answers. He doesn't expect us to know what he knows, but to trust that all things he designs or permits are for our good, if we will but follow his voice. And that is often a hard lesson to learn. His thoughts are not our thoughts, nor are his ways our ways. They are far beyond any wisdom we might think we have. Joe tried to match wits with God. In his early years he had a smattering of religious instruction in Europe, but its effect was soon lost when he came to America to make his fortune. And make it he did! Who needs God when all goes well? He was a craftsman of great abilities, easily found profitable employment, and within just a few short years was able to buy a half-interest in the corporation he worked for.

He married, and the union was blessed with a healthy daughter. He bought a good home, had all the things the family wanted, and put aside enough to give him a strong sense of security. For almost fifteen years, nothing happened to spoil his dream of the good life.

Joe went to the doctor's office one day for his annual physical checkup. He hadn't been feeling too well, and some of the old drive had departed. But that did not trouble him, until the doctor suggested indepth tests at a hospital, to study a shadow in the lung X-ray. Later, at the hospital, Joe received the shock of his optimistic life: "You have an infection in your lung, very contagious, and it can be treated only in a specialty sanatorium. It may take months; it may take years, before you can resume former activities!" (This happened before the discovery of "miracle medications" that now control tuberculosis.)

Shock wave number two: Joe's wife died very suddenly of unrecognized causes, and now the heavy responsibilities of raising a sixteen-year-old daughter fell solely upon him. And shock wave number three: laboratory tests confirmed that Joe had infected his daughter with his disease, and she too had to be hospitalized in isolation!

Joe's world had fallen apart. How were the pieces to be put together again? He was never a quitter, and mainly for his daughter's sake he began to fight back. He soon found, though, that Coueism ("day by day I'm getting better and better") and all other human philosophies were of little or no help.

His former business partner called on him often. He was a Christian through and through and lived his faith as an example to all. Naturally, he often spoke with Joe about God and the many satisfactions and strengths God provided for us pilgrims, as we wind our way through this life, so spoiled by the sins of all. In short, as often as could be done without antagonizing Joe, he spoke about the Savior and the hope he alone could create in fallen man. He also encouraged Joe and his daughter to attend the Lutheran services held there each week in the Chapel of Good Hope.

Before, it had been all work, clothes, food, house, and pleasure. Now came a reevaluation of man's life and destiny. "What good is it for someone to gain the whole world, yet forfeit their soul?" (Mark 8:36). This question was intriguing. The answer could come only from God. And it did come.

At first, Joe listened to our services via the bed phone broadcast. Then he invited his daughter to do the same. And soon, when the staff permitted them to attend, both joined us on service nights to hear the appealing voice of the Good Shepherd. We had visited a number of times previously, but the visits were somewhat stand-offish as though Joe feared any closer relationship might draw him into something he wasn't ready for.

But, as I found later, it was the daughter who suggested that they sit down in earnest to study God's part in man's life. Joe was willing. Formal instructions began, and over the course of several months we met twice a week, the three of us, to talk about God and his Word. Through all of our talks ran a golden thread, our Maker's supernatural love in sending us a Shepherd to lead and guide us through the maze of our earthly sojourn. It seems there was no end to new discoveries of the real meaning of life and the proper understanding of our reverses and sufferings.

What a happy night it was when this man and his daughter "joined" our Good Hope congregation at the San! In that night's chapel services, they sincerely professed their faith and spoke their vows. The daughter was baptized, and both of them received the sacrament of Holy Communion for the first time. The whole group of worshipers joined in thanking a gracious God for having rescued two more sheep from the spiritual wolves bent on their destruction.

The father has, since that day, entered his eternal home in the mansions of God. The daughter has recovered from her disease and by God's help lives to await a happy reunion.

SOLVING LIFE'S MYSTERIES

"Peace I leave with you; my peace I give you. I do not give to you as the world gives. Do not let your hearts be troubled and do not be afraid" (John 14:27).

Much is said and written today about peace of mind, peace of soul. Someone has said that if you want to write a bestseller, just promise people inner peace and calmness of soul in the struggle of life. Bookstore sales will verify this contention. Strange, isn't it, that people will seek peace apart from him who alone can give it?

Marie was a patient at the Sanatorium mentioned earlier. Beautiful and very fragile, she lost her health by being led astray by a man-about-town husband whose god was much money, good times, much drinking and carousing, and the wrong kind of friends. She followed his lead with exuberance, because his ways seemed to put a great deal of spice into life. Zesty and full of fun, she was really living! Her two growing sons were no problem—they were being raised by substitute parents, grandpa and grandma, while she was free to follow her inclinations and desires. Life seemed to keep her pantry well supplied, until the day that tragedy struck. It came in the form of bad news from her doctor that her growing frailness and loss of weight were due to an advanced stage of tuberculosis, a dreadful, consuming disease that so slyly invaded the system and gave little hope of recovery.

Shortly before she entered the San, her high-flying husband had deserted her and her boys, mainly because of her inability to keep up with him in his fast pace. She had to move back to her parental home and become a dependent. And now, more trouble; she faced the prospect of a long stay in that foreboding 650-bed Sanatorium.

Every minor sign of improvement in her condition brought renewed hope for complete recovery. But each such sign was followed by further distressing developments in her debilitating lung disease. She couldn't help noticing the weekly loss of weight, the increasing shortness of breath, and the frequency of chest pains. She became convinced that she was going to die.

There had been a time in her life when she had been taught something about God and his Shepherd-Son, but she didn't pay much attention to it, because for her, the tangible things had always been so much more exciting. Now in a period of crisis, however, her thoughts turned to God, to judgment, and to eternity. She began to devour religious literature, such as Science and Health by Mary Baker Eddy, and other books that attempted to tell the truth about life and death. For a time, she thought that her newly found mind-over-matter approach was bringing peace to her troubled soul. But she soon discovered that trying to deny the reality of her desperate physical condition was no comfort at all. It only sharpened her awareness of daily deterioration.

Then some friends led her into the beliefs and practices of Catholicism. On the advice of a priest, she threw herself into a fervent round of pious acts and prayers. She was sincerely seeking to appease and please a God she knew hated sin and pronounced eternal condemnation upon transgressors. The more she tried to please him and find peace in his approbation, the more she became discouraged by the lack of perfection she found in herself. There was no real peace in her soul or trust in God's compassion and free forgiveness. This, added to her concern for her aging parents and for the future of her two boys, made each day a fearful ordeal for all. She gave up Catholicism.

During the many months that these things were happening to Marie, I often stopped at her bedside while making rounds in her ward. As I visited and ministered to some of our Lutheran patients, invariably, she overheard our conversations. I also stopped at her bed to wish her well and to point her to some word of Scripture, which directed man to see not only his damning sin, but especially God's limitless and unconditional relief from its ravages through our Mediator, the Shepherd Jesus Christ. She seemed to appreciate that and always thanked me for the effort to help her find peace.

Finally one day came her weak request: "Would you have time to teach me more about your Lutheran religion? How can I be sure of being saved?" I assured her that I would comply with her wishes and immediately begin a course of instruction in the basics of Christian truth, using the Bible and Catechism as textbooks. The sessions had to be short, simple, and frequent, because time was running out very fast for Marie. Over a period of several weeks, we managed to cover all she needed to know for her salvation. What a satisfaction it was to see how the Holy Spirit filled her heart with understanding and firm acceptance of God's love! And she herself, without any urging from me, declared her willingness for confirmation. She wanted to be a member of our church.

Only a few nights later, before we were able to confirm her formally, I received a call from the night nurse telling me that Marie's condition had suddenly turned critical, and that she was asking to see me. It was late, about 11:00 p.m., when I arrived. Marie had been moved to the special room near the nurses' station, a room reserved for the critical and dying. Her parents came at about the same time and heard her request to be confirmed in their presence. "Tonight," she said, "Please, tonight."

It was not that she was afraid to die, but because she wanted them to know how she trusted the Good Shepherd to lead her to the green pastures and still waters beyond the valley of the shadow. I'm sure she also wanted them to absorb the meaning of dying as a victor rather than a victim.

I excused myself for a few moments to quickly scribble out our form for the Rite of Confirmation from the Agenda and to give the parents time to talk with their daughter at this most tender time. When I returned to the room, there were tear-filled eyes. Marie's tears were an expression of gratitude, as they washed away every stain of sin through the precious cleansing of the Shepherd's blood, the parents' tears—who can possibly describe the anguish of a good father or mother watching their child die?

We asked Marie the usual questions about her faith and also her intent to abide in that confession. In firm voice she answered, the voice of solid conviction. You just couldn't help being deeply impressed by her sincerity and spirit of relief from a heavy burden. That was particularly noticeable as she received the body and blood of her slain Savior. "Given and shed for you for the remission of all your sins," we said. Her heart responded, "Yes, for me."

About an hour later Marie's soul was carried by the angels to "Abraham's bosom," never again to know problems or pains. And a few days later, we buried her corruptible body in God's earth, to await the trumpet call on the Last Day to rise again and live with our Shepherd forever.

The final outcome of Marie's "triumphant tragedy" was that her people returned to their long-neglected church, brought up her boys, had them instructed and confirmed, and lived to see them become valuable assets to the church and society. Memories of the past may bring a few tears now and then. Yet they are the kind of tears that are wholesome, because they reflect the kindnesses and mercies of the Good Shepherd who shed his blood that angels might sing when one lost sheep is returned to the flock.

FAITHFUL FRANK

"Whom have I in heaven but you? And earth has nothing I desire besides you. My flesh and my heart may fail, but God is the strength of my heart and my portion forever" (Psalm 73:25, 26).

This confession of the Psalmist might well have been painted on the cracked plaster walls of Frank's ten-by-ten foot room at the County Infirmary. They were a publicly demonstrated statement of his philosophy of life.

He had been born in something less than a normal and desirable home and had been ill most of his life. After his family had died, he had to shift for himself and make his way with the occasional aid of some friends. Soon these also disappeared, leaving Frank all alone.

A diabetic condition developed together with his many other physical problems, and when he left the hospital he was minus both legs. They had to be amputated above the knees. What now? He was helpless! His only option for shelter and care was to become a ward of public charity and live in the county infirmary. The adjustment to this new life was not easy by any means, but Frank had no second choice, and so he made the best of it.

The daily routine was depressing, of course. Attendants had to bathe and dress him every morning and then help him into his wheelchair where he spent the day. He took his meals in a large dining room, which served about 300 at a setting. The waiters were ambulatory fellow patients. When the evening meal was over, he was helped into his bed to lie there for hours reminiscing until sleep finally took over.

While Frank was at the Infirmary, he met the Lutheran missionary pastor and became interested in God's story of life and eternity. Before long, he was being instructed in the fundamentals of Biblical truth and later was confirmed and became a communicant. Any visitor from the outside who attended our services in the second floor chapel couldn't help noticing him as he sat in his wheelchair just to one side of the altar Sunday after Sunday. There was good reason for him to occupy that spot, for on Communion Sundays, it facilitated his reception of the sacrament at the altar step. Rarely, unless ill, did this man miss a service.

But his deeply-rooted dedication to his Lord was shown also in the manner by which he laboriously made his way to the chapel from the first floor. There were no elevators in this oldest building on the county compound. In his chair, he would wheel himself to the bottom step of the two-flight stairway leading to the chapel. Once at the step, he would reach into a small box attached to his chair and take out a pair of white canvas gloves to cover his hands. Then, with much effort, he would edge out of the chair, crawl to the first step and with difficulty make his way upwards to the second floor.

Meanwhile, aides or volunteers would carry his chair up the steps, so that it would be ready for him to use in proceeding to the chapel area. Once at the top, he would again ease himself into the chair, remove his gloves and roll on to the services. After the services were ended, the whole procedure would be repeated until he arrived in his room. This action, recurring so often in his many years at the Infirmary, was a powerful lesson to all who saw it, especially to many of the indifferent inmates who usually stood around in idleness in the main corridor.

It wouldn't surprise us at all to hear that many people today remember our friend Frank, particularly the people who attended school at St. John's in Wauwatosa. For more than forty years, St. John's schoolchildren repeated their annual Christmas program on the afternoon of December 25, for the joy of the fifty or more aged people who made up our congregation at the Infirmary. What a real Christmas Day for these aged and lonely people! To see children and to hear them sing and speak of the newborn Savior was a thrilling experience some of them kept mentioning for weeks after. Lambs of the flock were helping tend the weak older sheep!

For Frank and for many others, the Psalmist's motto took on intensified meaning: "Whom have I in heaven but you? And earth has nothing I desire besides you" (Psalm 73:25).

THE MYSTERY OF GOD'S LOVE

"He tends his flock like a shepherd: He gathers the lambs in his arms and carries them close to his heart" (Isaiah 40:11).

It was early evening when the hospital desk called with the emergency message that a young child was critically ill and not expected to live long. The parents were there and, having no clergyman of their own, happily accepted the offer of the charge nurse to call a chaplain who could advise and help them.

This is the scene outside the child's room: The parents, of course, were upset and apprehensive. In their church, not Lutheran, infant baptism was not taught as a means of grace for small children; rather, it was frowned upon as "an unreasonable belief." In it also they found little to attract them to the Word of God, and so some time ago they let their membership lapse and became unchurched. That all added to their feeling of helplessness as they stood at the bedside watching their youngest die. What can we do? Where can we turn? The offer of the nurse was most welcome.

Because they were not at all sure that they were doing everything they could in their spiritual responsibility to God and their child, they were most agreeable to listen to what the Bible says about parents and their duties to the children the Lord places under their care. And, after we had briefly reviewed what baptism is and does, they asked me to perform the sacred act for their child. I did.

That night the little one died, and the next day the parents asked me to conduct the burial service at a funeral home. It was a privilege to speak on that occasion about a common need of mankind for a shepherd, who can lead us securely through the labyrinth of this world, to the mansions he has created in timeless eternity. Even little children, under the curse of sin from birth because they are born of sinful flesh, need to be washed clean of all guilt. In his grace, God gave us the sacrament of baptism to provide that cleansing, create faith, and begin the work of regeneration. There was honest comfort for these parents as they placed their little one into the grave.

The Word surely was having its effect, as we learned shortly after the committal at the cemetery, when the parents solemnly approached me with another plea for assistance. There were three other children in the family, none of them baptized. Would I come to their home soon "to make them children of God?"

Again, I was happy to oblige. On a Sunday afternoon I went to their house where there was much more poverty than possessions. But it was a clean house with well-behaved children, who welcomed me as an old friend. They seemed to understand quite well what happened to their little brother, and they wanted the same to happen to them.

Briefly I again explained the rudiments of the sacrament. It was not some magical act, but the beginning of a new life in the promises of the Word. We ought to hear it, believe it, and obey it. They promised that by God's grace it would be so. And by the things they said and the way they conducted themselves, they showed that they knew something divine had happened to them. They were happy, and so were their parents.

The story did not end there, and probably is not ended to this day. The parents became interested in enrolling their children in both day and Sunday school, and with the cooperation of a neighboring pastor of our church, arrangements were made to fulfill their desire. What about father and mother? Voluntarily, they joined the pastor's adult instruction class, and eventually were accepted into membership in his congregation!

Months later the mailman brought a note from that family. It was filled with words of gratitude for having helped them find true peace in a situation that might well have returned often to haunt them with thoughts of neglect and self-condemnation. We responded with words of encouragement to faithfulness. And we prayed that the Good Shepherd, who had taken their child into his bosom, would guard and protect them and bring all of them one day into his flock in heaven.

PRAYER ANSWERED IN A STRANGE WAY

"And we know that in all things God works for the good of those who love him, who have been called according to his purpose" (Romans 8:28).

Some very strange things occur in the life of a hospital pastor. Here and there the sequence of events spins a tale that is almost incredible. But as we review the step-by-step happenings, we see God's mighty hand working before our eyes to verify the Bible truth expressed above.

A man collapsed and was rushed to the Medical Complex one night. The first quick diagnosis by the attending physician already placed him on the critical list, and when the sustaining staff got into action, there was no longer any question about it; the man was going to die. Since his admission sheet in the chart did not list any religion, I was called to his bedside to minister to him.

Unlike many other patients, this man was surprisingly well-versed in Bible knowledge. He knew he was a sinner in need of

God's pardon. He was aware of the seriousness of his illness and the possibility that he might soon die. And, though somewhat shakily, he confessed that his one hope was in the Lamb of God. He trusted, so he said, that if he died, God would receive his soul and grant him the joys of heaven.

That kind of patient is easy to work with at the time of death, because of his reliance on the Word. We talked about it quite a bit, and when we had finished for the time being, he asked me to pray also for God's protection and care for his wife and children. This I gladly did. As I left the hospital that night, I thanked my Lord for the privilege of helping such a one in a time of crisis.

What I kept thinking about was the fact that he was not a member of any church, yet so well informed in Christian faith and life. He had told me that his wife and children were faithful in school and church at one of our Lutheran congregations. Yet he had so often refused to go with them, because he was of another religious background that was incompatible with the family's practices. Besides, he did not want to alienate his father and mother entirely by turning to his wife's faith. This arrangement made the family sad, the man's parents disagreeable, and the patient miserable!

He also told me that every Sunday, while the family was at church, he would spend time in the bedroom reading his wife's Bible and personal prayer book. That accounted for his knowledge of truth. He was hearing the Good Shepherd's voice and responding to it in his heart. And when we were informed that he died that night, we were happy that another sheep (though secretly a sheep) had been relieved of all ills in this life and the next.

While talking with a fellow pastor later that morning by telephone, he told me that he had had a sad experience earlier, when one of his loyal members had come to his study weeping over the death of her husband the previous night. She knew he was a good man, but she was fearful for his salvation; he had been stubborn about openly professing his religious views. The pastor tried to give her what little comfort he could under the circumstances, but had to refuse her tearful request to officiate at the funeral services.

As the pastor spoke, my mind went back to the man I had ministered to at the hospital the past evening. A light went on! I asked the name of the parishioner and, would you believe it, it was the name of the man I had served. The pastor hurried to the woman's home and then brought her to mine. It was a wonderful half-hour we spent together: me telling her of the staunch confession of sin and forgiveness through Jesus that I heard from her dying husband's lips, and she telling me of the joy she never expected to know, in spite of her many hearty prayers for her husband's redemption. Joy! Joy in the midst of earthly grief, because the Shepherd was hearing all the time and working things out for the good of his sheep.

Two days later we had a burial service for the deceased. Mainly because it was during the Lenten season, I chose as the text for the sermon the story of the thief on the cross who had turned to Jesus in his dying moments and had heard the blessed words: "Truly I tell you, today you will be with me in paradise." (Luke 23:43).

A good many Christians might resent such a text used at the burial of their loved one, but not this knowing and devoted wife. She later wrote a letter, in which she expressed thankfulness for the comfort she and her children drew from that particular Word of God in their time of sorrow! ALL things had worked for good!

PEACE THAT MONEY CANNOT BUY

"Call upon me in the day of trouble; I will deliver you, and you will honor me" (Psalm 50:15).

An anonymous phone call led me to a certain room in a local hospital. The details given me by the caller were very scanty, but enough to make an entry into this stranger's life easy and smooth. It was one of the more lavishly appointed rooms, and a private nurse was on duty. All seemed to indicate that here was a man of means who could afford the best of anything, the type one does not usually find in our special ministry. But as we soon found out, there was something essential lacking, something that a world of material wealth could never supply.

The patient was in critical condition, terminally ill. He appeared pleased with the call and anxious to converse with a pastor. He told me how he had been active in his church for many years, but then had left the church because it did not tolerate membership in godless lodges. It was a policy of his business corporation that all of its executives acquire such memberships for the promotion of its interests and the prestige of its top officers.

Faced with the choice of mediocre living or great plenty, the man chose the latter and after a time became comfortable in it. Then, when his church declared him ineligible for Holy Communion, his conscience pinched a bit, but soon was stilled by the compensations of his affluent living. Besides, he had married a woman of another faith. Since she was not insistent on his participation in church affairs, he soon fell into a state of indifference and complacency.

Years went by, and living was rich and good. Up, up, and up he climbed on the ladder to success, and soon he was at the top, breathing the rarefied air of the rich man in Jesus' parable who said, "What shall I do? I have no place to store my crops" (Luke 12:17). Seemingly there was nothing that could ever spoil his satisfactions.

There came that day at the office, however, when stabbing stomach pains sent him scurrying to the doctor's office and then to the hospital. It was thought that he was suffering from the ordinary "successful businessman's ulcer," but in a few days the doctors were concerned about their inability to control Mr. Jones' pain. A series of tests and repeated X-rays brought the studied diagnosis: "A serious cardiac condition, complicated by a rapidly-growing cancer."

The props of our patient's powerful world suddenly collapsed completely. Why this? What now? There must be some help! Get the best specialists, for there must be something they could do to restore health and preserve life.

No, you must die and face your Maker! Jesus said the same in other words in the story referred to above: "You fool! This very night your life will be demanded from you. Then who will get what you have prepared for yourself? This is how it will be with anyone who stores up things for himself but is not rich toward God."

A close friend had noted Mr. Jones' extreme agitation. Sensing that a major part of the problem was spiritual, this friend had made a phone call to an institutional missionary.

How relieved Mr. Jones was when he could share his chief burden with a pastor! He spoke about his past as a confessing child of God. He could not and did not deny the antichristian spirit and teachings of the lodge. Over and over he told me how sorry he was for having been blinded by temptations to "the good life." He was like a little child, unquestioningly accepting the truths of the Word and clinging desperately to its promises. And that's when the Good Shepherd can truly comfort and guide one of his sheep.

Many times over in our daily visits he would humbly ask, "Can God really forgive me?" The remorse and shame of his acquired habit of despising God's Word in worship and Communion was a tool Satan now used to confuse and create doubt in his last attempts to steal this sheep from the fold. And every assurance from Scripture, about the unconditional pardon offered any sinner by the blood of Jesus, seeped into his soul like water disappearing into hot desert sands.

Early one evening I met his wife weeping at the closed door to Mr. Jones' room. She was upset by a problem. That day a letter addressed to her husband had arrived at their home. The envelope told her that it was a communication from her husband's lodge. Among themselves they had agreed not to open each other's mail, and she didn't want to break that agreement. Yet she felt that this might be something important, and that she should open it. Incidentally, she was never in sympathy with his fraternal connection. She considered it to be morally wrong and hypocritical in effect.

Under the circumstances, I advised her to open the letter and read it. When she did, both of us were pleasantly surprised at its contents: A release from the Order! We learned later, that with the help of a nurse, Mr. Jones had, under great difficulty, written his request for the release, "Because it was the only right thing to do."

Less than a week later, the man died peacefully in his sleep. The services were held with many men, giants in industry, attending. What do you say on such an occasion to people who considered this death an irretrievable loss? Nothing but God's truth: That ALL men must die and face the judgment of an omniscient God. Big men, little men, rich men, poor men, ALL will stand before the court of absolute justice one day. How happy and safe are those who know the Shepherd and follow him to eternal bliss!

MENTALLY AND EMOTIONALLY SICK SHEEP

Humanly speaking, one of the saddest and most self-effacing illnesses that afflict people is the derangement of the mind. For one reason or another the brain does not function normally, and the patient lapses temporarily or permanently into a world of unreality and delusions. Some are born that way; others suffer brain injuries by disease or accident. Whatever the case, life becomes subnormal or abnormal and too often results in segregation from family, friends, and church.

Not many years ago we had a long list of categories attempting to define mental health or illness, but more recent medical viewpoints tend to simplify diagnoses and treat most cases with drug therapies. The greatest challenge to medical science appears to be the emotional disorders that defy the skills of experts in the field. Then too there are the puzzling psychosomatic cases in which the mind and behavior is affected by physical ills and/or the body functions are impaired by aberrations in the mind. In either case, the sickness is real and most disturbing to the patient and his loved ones.

Because our purpose is to exalt the power of the Word, we will avoid the trap of posing as medical, psychiatric, or psychological experts in this area of man's sufferings. Only as undershepherds on the staff of the great Physician will we seek to understand and ease the woe of a sheep so afflicted. Jesus never shied away from those who were looked upon as being "different" and neither should we. We have a "therapy" for them: the reassurance of God's love and help.

In the ministry of an institutional pastor, dealing with abnormalities among the sheep becomes rather commonplace.

Whether it is in the Diagnostic Center or the Mental Health Center for acute or chronic cases, or especially in working with children's behavioral problems, he meets head-on with pitiful sights and heart-touching pleas for help. Though he may often feel helpless in responding to the patients' needs, he is constantly mindful that his privilege is to sow the seeds of the simple Word of truth on every occasion, leaving the production of the fruits to the Master.

And those fruits are produced by him to the amazement of doctors, pastors, and families. We might call the whole process "faith-healing," but not in the sense that the public often understands this term today. We have no "holy places" where people with broken limbs go to pray and then throw away their crutches. We have no "shrines" where miracles are expected. We do have the Word which, in the power of God's choosing, does what he commands.

Each of our mental health hospitals provides ample space for religious services in a well-appointed chapel. Administrators and staff may not look upon church activities in the same light as we do, but they realize there is a value in worship and prayer in the lives of individuals and use this to assist in treating the patients. When we were operating at capacity (1100 patients in one psychiatric hospital and 2300 in another), about 100 would voluntarily "go to church" on Sunday morning. It was a rare thing to have any kind of disturbance during the worship, and many would thank the pastor for the hymns they enjoyed singing and the sermons they listened to so devoutly. On special days a visiting choir would make the attendees feel that the outside world really cared for them and put forth extra effort to serve them. All this helped create a confidence in the "chaplain" that made them ready for personal visitation with him.

SHAME OVERCOME

This was demonstrated one day on a ward of some sixty women patients. The ward doctor wanted to experiment on a woman with the use of sodium-amytal, a drug new at the time and often referred to as "truth serum." It completely relaxed a patient so that he or she was supposed to reveal deep inner thoughts when under its influence. He could not prevail on the woman to submit to this treatment. She would rather suffer her condition of uncontrollable bad behavior. That's why she was in the hospital; she could not be trusted to do right at home or among people generally.

Her doctor asked me if I would help by encouraging her to accept his advice, and then while under the influence of the drug speak to her as I would speak to any other patient. It was his hope that she might open a secret door to her mind, ventilate her inner feelings, and give some clue for future treatment. She consented to cooperate when told that I would be at her side.

She was given the drug and shortly thereafter I began to speak with her about many things concerning God. We spoke about the Commandments and our failure to keep them. And she was well aware of punishment and condemnation. We also spoke at length about Jesus, through whom it is possible for us to believe God's promises of forgiveness. She knew these things but became agitated at any reminder of our guilt.

Suddenly, and quite unexpectedly, she began to cry softly and then sob almost convulsively. When she stopped sobbing, she began to speak with muted voice. She was confessing a sin of unfaithfulness against her husband many years ago, a terrible sin she had never repeated. But locking it up in her heart had hurt; she could tell no one—only think about her shame. The situation had overpowered her so that she could no longer function as a "normal" person.

Once again assuring her of God's grace always being greater than our sin, and speaking a prayer that our merciful God would relieve the conscience of this disturbed woman, I left the room.

The following week, while on that ward visiting patients, I chanced on the doctor involved in the amytal case. I asked how our patient was and where I might find her. To my utter amazement he replied, "Oh, haven't you heard? She was discharged over the weekend and returned to her family." Cured! By what? The drug? My prayer? No, simply by the Word of God's revelation, the trust to believe that overcame the temptation to doubt.

For special reasons, the drug method is not in wide use. We often wonder what the results might be if it were. If it would help lead one disturbed sheep back to mental health, all of us would be grateful and happy.

TRUTH STRANGER THAN FICTION

Almost as "sensational" was my experience with Lydia in the chronic division of the Mental Health Center. She was very irrational, and because of her violent flare-ups few people wanted anything to do with her,

I frankly admit that it was often an undesirable duty to stop at the small room in which she was confined, to see her shackled to her bed to protect her from danger she might do to herself. Yet, since the family and her pastor had asked me to visit her when I was in that building, I tried every way I knew to get her to be quiet for a few minutes and listen to the Word. Time after time I was disappointed and left her room in defeat.

Lydia was a chronic case who seemed unapproachable in her outbursts. She had come from a devout Lutheran family, well-informed in Christian doctrine and practice, and dedicated completely to the service of the Lord. From teen years on into middle age, she had given many years to the Shepherd and his flock in teaching Sunday school and doing secretarial work for the congregation. I'm sure many a lamb learned to recognize the Shepherd's voice and to follow him through the efforts of this woman.

She became ill, very ill, and most likely the prolonged high fever had something to do with the damage her brain suffered. And when her mother could no longer manage her at home, she had to be placed in custodial care at what was then named the Asylum. This was done with great reluctance and in sadness. After all, the parents and brothers and sisters loved their own flesh and blood and were heartbroken at her plight.

Can we possibly imagine their sorrow when they visited her several times a week, only to hear foul cursings and vile talk? To see her tied to her bed? To know that she was so out of touch with reality that she didn't know them? That's a real test of faith in the mercies of God! For years her lips had spoken many blessings; now they pronounced revilings and smut the family did not want to hear.

One day at her bedside I sadly listened to her rantings for a while and then, taking her hand, tried to break in with some choice gems of Scripture, hoping that some word or phrase might be recognized by her as God speaking to her. It appeared to be another hopeless effort. But after a few minutes of out shouting her, Lydia became more and more quiet, as though she were listening and straining to hear.

That spark of hope disappeared in a hurry when she turned her head to the wall while I prayed for God's mercy on her soul. Even the Lord's Prayer brought no response.

As I quietly and dejectedly left her room, just before I closed the door I heard a weak call, "Pastor, will you come again?" I went back in but could rouse no further conversation. I did spend a few moments, however, to tell her that I would return soon and that we would read more of her Good Shepherd's words from the Bible. She was assured that God's mighty love and the Savior's compassion were with her in this time of severe testing.

Well, it is hard to believe, but it is true—we, the relatives and I, never again heard a word of cursing from her! She accepted her sickness as a part of God's plan for her life and resigned herself to his superior wisdom in those few more months she had to suffer on earth. Valiantly she bore her cross in the footsteps of her Savior.

To be sure, none of us has any right to feel that we can by our own techniques become "miracle workers" or expect the unusual to happen every time we apply the Word to a problem case. But, at the same time, we should never hesitate or stop using the Word of God, even when all seems hopeless. We never know what God may want to accomplish through it.

YOUTHFUL DILEMMA

Is it possible to "get too much religion"? If one learns a smattering of many different religious teachings, one could easily end up being very confused about truth, or half-truth, or spurious truth. And if a child is subjected to such a variety and dubious mixtures, it is easy to understand that there could be a serious mental breakdown at an early age. An elderly doctor friend contacted me to ask a favor. He was upset about his grandson who had been institutionalized in a mental health hospital. The best of psychiatrists were trying to help him to normalcy, but they were stymied by some deep-seated psychosis, and no progress was being made. There were evidences that the boy's religious misun-derstandings played a strong role in twisting his mind and directing his bizarre behavior.

Biff, as they called him, was the son of a United Nations employee whose duties took him and his family all over the world on special assignments. They would be in one place for about three months and then move on to another, sometimes thousands of miles away. No wonder it was such a task to educate and train the children, a responsibility that rested particularly on the young mother. Since the family had religious roots, the children became familiar with many general Protestant denominations, and some-times in isolated areas of the world the parents sent them to whatever church was there. Biff, a super-intelligent boy, absorbed a little of anything and everything. Whatever church you named, he could tell you something about its profession and way of life.

While the family was in Korea on a mission, the parents noticed signs of very strange behavior in Biff and consequently arranged to send him back to America to become readjusted in the home of his grandfather. And that is where his problems really broke out in force. The concerned grandfather asked me for help.

The boy was about fourteen years old, and his hospitali-zation tended to add to his confusion and cause him to withdraw into a world of his own. It was so difficult for the staff to deal with his case because he would not speak, not even to his grand-father, whom he had loved dearly. About the first four or five times I tried visiting him, he would not respond to any questions nor comment on anything I said.

Then one day after I entered his locked ward, I saw him dart around a corner to the end of the long corridor, as though he wanted to hide from me. Quietly I made my way around the same corner and found Biff in the bathroom. He was busy at the sink, washing the pages of a Bible. After watching him for a short time, I asked why he was washing God's Book. There was no answer, but he had a guilty look on his face and acted as though he was afraid he might be punished.

He followed my invitation to go to his room and talk about the God who had written that Book. No one was more surprised than I at his willingness to talk that afternoon. First we talked generally about the Scriptures, and then we tried to lead him into the purpose of that monumental work, namely, to have sinners know and believe in Jesus as the one who died on a cross to satisfy God's just claims on us.

Biff's eyes began to shine, and for the first time since I had gotten to know him he smiled briefly, as though he wanted to indicate that this was good news for him. We had, of course, talked about the good news of salvation several times earlier, but with no response. This conversation seemed to be a breakthrough, though, that we hadn't dared to hope for before.

At the end of the visit as he walked with me to the ward door, I "jumped in with both feet" and bluntly asked him why he had been washing his Bible with soap and water. In a moment he told me. Every time he read God's Book, he felt guilty and unacceptable. Every religion he had learned previously, or snatches of it, told him about the Commandments and how he had broken every one. The pages I had referred to him for reading became a gift for others, but not for him. The gospel was for the good, not the sinning. And he had come to feel so dirty in the sight of God that he tried to wash away the words that reminded him of his guilt.

From that day on it was always a pleasure to visit Biff. He learned to pray properly and humbly in Jesus' name. Every day, before reading some portion of the Word, he would ask the Holy Spirit to lead him to all truth and make his day happy as he walked with the Good Shepherd. Many passages of promise he memorized and was happy to repeat in my presence.

In consultation with his advisors, I revealed my experiences with Biff. They were grateful, because they could chart his improvement daily. They even labeled his mental illness with some fancy name I have long forgotten. But I will never forget him and what the Word of God did for him in its power to turn sinners into saints.

I don't know where Biff may be today. I lost contact with him after he left the hospital and rejoined his family. The grandfather is dead. The mother wrote once from Europe to express thanks for our services, and I had a brief phone conversation with her after grandfather's funeral. She was at the airport, ready to fly off to Africa.

The one thing I hope is that the Shepherd's voice may always be clear to Biff in whatever career he may have chosen for his life's usefulness.

WITH GOD NOTHING IS IMPOSSIBLE

Our hearts go out to those children who are born with radical physical defects. We also suffer with those whose physical bodies are normal but the development of the mental faculties lags behind. How parents must anguish when they see their little one grow up under all such difficult consequences!

We meet many such patients in public institutions. One I find especially hard to forget. I would like to share her story, as a measure of hope, for those who fear that their loved one may never understand the love and forgiving grace of the Shepherd Jesus, and thus be deprived of the joys of heaven.

This young girl was separated from her parents and home by placement into a Lutheran Home miles away: It was hoped that every known treatment and technique available would help the girl to understand the basics of God's revealed truth and help her know and love her Savior. After several years Elsie had mastered the Creed and the Lord's Prayer, and that seemed to be the crest of her capabilities.

When the Home could no longer control her behavior, she was transferred to a public mental health center-chronic division. There she was placed in a large ward for custodial care. She was considered to be a hopeless case consigned to live the rest of her life in what one writer calls the "snake pit." And that is where we first met her when she was about sixteen years old.

Elsie's top-grade Christian family had told me the story of her past and stated that they did not expect me to spend much time with her "because all that could be done has been done. We place her into our Lord's compassionate care." However, though she appeared to be oblivious of my presence when I spoke to her on my visits to that ward, I never left her without speaking a word of promise or hope from our God. The simplest of prayers and hymn verses were repeated for her. All seemed to be so fruitless, yet it was the least we could do for this poor soul. And this went on for years.

One Sunday morning we were surprised and stunned to see Elsie in chapel among some seventy or eighty other worshipers. We watched her closely during the service, partly out of wonderment at her presence and partly because we feared that she might cause some disturbance. But as she sat through the worship, she was quiet. In fact, she gave no signs of comprehension. She was there in body, but in spirit too? We wondered why the aides had taken the trouble to dress her and bring her along with others from that ward. Sunday after Sunday now Elsie "went to church." Why? Out of an acquired mechanical habit? Or because some kind ward attendant invited her? We were especially puzzled because, in every service, she fixed her eyes on the ceiling and only participated when we would repeat the words of the Creed or Lord's Prayer.

Late one night the real test came. I was called by the night supervisor and told that Elsie had been put into the hospital ward because of a bad case of pneumonia. She was critically ill. (It was routine policy of the institution to call a chaplain any hour of day or night whenever one of his patient's lives was in jeopardy.) Under the circumstances in this case, can you imagine how heavy my feet were as I walked down that long and quiet corridor to the "death room"? What could I do to help her dispel the shadow in the valley of death? What could I say? Praying for the Master's guidance, I entered the room. Only he could truly help.

This was in the Advent season, close to Christmas. So I sat down at her bedside and began the ministration with a simple telling of the happiness that the Christchild brought to our world of sin and suffering; how he came out of love for unworthy sheep who had left his fold; how by his keeping of the law and his death on the cross the gate to the sheepfold was opened again to us, that we might live forever with him in heaven.

Several times Elsie opened her eyes briefly, and several times would utter single, simple words and short phrases. She knew the story of Christmas! Her words became louder and understandable. She was trying to tell the story in her own childlike way. I asked her direct questions and received confessing answers. And, when I later began to pray the Lord's Prayer, she joined in and completed it to the end.

What a happy trip it was back home that cold and snowy night! The angels in heaven were singing God's praises and the stars brightly proclaimed: "Jesus is the light of the world." Powerful light he is, stronger than any human scientific creation, light that penetrates the darkness of human frailty and misery!

Elsie died that night. She went to heaven's Bethlehem to rejoice with all saints over him who became poor, that we might be forever rich.

So unusual was our experience with this helpless patient that the family found the story hard to believe. It took a quick trip to the hospital that day and a visit with the nurse who had been with me at Elsie's bedside to reassure them. Later we could join them in repeated expressions of gratitude to our Good Shepherd.

Elsie's funeral service days later was truly a happy service of thanksgiving. For all of us it was a time of rededication to the service of the Word among people. And may it ever be a lifetime of greater trust in our Shepherd's leading!

AN ORPHANS'S PLIGHT

Many times life becomes so complicated by reverses and unfulfilled desires that the mind becomes boggled by the daily pressures and gradually loses its sense of good direction. Not all people have equal strengths to bear their crosses patiently, and as they become emotionally involved to a high pitch, they are led to do strange things, wrong things. Some become psychopathic personalities.

A boy was adopted by a loving Lutheran family. He was just a baby when he entered their home, and they treated him as their own flesh and blood. In growing up, he had all the advantages of parochial school and a Lutheran high school. He was a normal and happy youth.

In conversation with one of his high school friends an argument arose, and Bob's friend struck a cruel blow by suggesting that Bob was adopted as an illegitimate child and therefore was something lesser than his schoolmates. Bob ignored the insinuation, but in the following days he thought about the possibility of the insinuations being true.

He spoke with his parents about the matter, but they tried to shield him from hurt by keeping the truth from him. Though well intended, their lack of openness was to have tragic consequences. Bob sensed that their evasiveness was a pretty sure indication that his friend at school was right in what he had said. The disturbance in his mind wouldn't go away, but grew as the days went by. Since the parents wouldn't or possibly couldn't tell Bob who his real father and mother were, he became perturbed to the point where his thoughts were constantly dwelling on the subject.

His school work suffered. There were interviews with faculty members and serious counseling sessions with the principal. They were all trying to help the troubled youth. But the attempts were ineffective. The obsession to know the facts of his life "threw him out of kilter." He quit school in his senior year and got a job. He worked diligently for long hours, earned good money, and put most of it aside in a savings account.

When he had saved quite a bit, he found a private detective agency that was willing to search for Bob's mother. They assigned a "private-eye" to the case, and he used all the resources at his command to locate the mysterious mother. He made trips to other cities on leads he thought might reveal who she was. And all this took money, much money. After some months Bob had to give up the search, because he could no longer afford it.

But the nagging pain in his mind and heart kept boring away within him. He moved to another city and found a real lucrative job. He soon established himself in a position of trust and became manager of considerable funds. I tended to believe him when he later told me that at first, as he was dipping into these funds in small sums, he had every intention of repaying all he was "borrowing." But the demands of the detective who was doing the new search soon were greater than Bob could manage.

From petty larceny he moved on to grand larceny, always able to cover his "loans" fictitiously. It was so until the auditors of the firm found evidence of Bob's illegal activities. When he was arrested for grand theft, he readily confessed and was sent to prison. What had been bad before became worse now. The many hours of loneliness and introspection did not diminish his desire to find his mother; they heightened his sense of frustration and self-defeat. Add to that the occasional twinges of the small inner voice, his conscience, and you have a picture of abject misery that just couldn't be painted out or glossed over. Mechanically, he went about his duties in the yard or shops of the prison compound, yet always hoping that someday he might know the truth of his parentage.

Bob's admission slip was given to me on one of my visits to the prison. I called him in for an interview to which he promptly responded. Maybe it was the accusation of conscience, maybe the trick of the devil, but the first few meetings between us did not give much promise in spiritual matters. But Bob did attend the chapel services and was an intent listener. The Shepherd was searching and calling a lost sheep.

Successive sessions with him brought out the whole story. I had to feel sorry for the young man, now in his early thirties. Our first objective was to have him realize his sins, how he had offended his gracious God by his many irresponsible actions. The second objective was to have him comforted by the pardon God alone can give, and the peace that can restore life to good balance and solid direction.

The Holy Spirit brought results. Bob was ashamed and truly sorry for his awful record of indifference to the Word during his major struggle in life. But he was also happy beyond words to have the Spirit unearth God's love in Christ from under all the rubble of wasted time and effort. He learned the lesson of being still and knowing that God was God. Strength came from Word and sacrament.

I don't really know how it happened, but soon after, he learned through the grapevine that a prison official's wife was his mother's sister! Once again the fires were stoked, and the possibility of finally knowing the truth of his birth occupied all his extra time and effort. I was his confidant by now and his contact with the warden. Through some legitimate maneuvering we managed a meeting between Bob and his aunt. She was the first blood relative he ever knew.

The aunt invested much money and many hours in tracing the family history. And she was successful!

But it would have been better if the revelation had remained hidden. Bob's mother was located in an apartment in one of our largest cities. When the sister found her, assisted by the authorities, she had been dead about two weeks. She had been a loose woman, kept for immoral purposes by many undesirable friends.

The shock to Bob and to his aunt had different effects, good and bad. For Bob the discovery was, in a sense, a tremendous relief. Though he now knew the awful truth, it served to help him thank God deeply for having been spared the terrible life known by his mother, and it drew him closer than ever to the sustaining arms of his Shepherd.

I wish the whole sordid story might have had some similar effect on Bob's aunt, but it didn't. She was so distraught and felt so disgraced. Even the gospel of forgiveness, the righting of all wrong things by a forgiving God, couldn't dent her soul at the time. She divorced her husband, moved far away, and only twice since then have I heard from her. Both times a phone call came at 2:00 A.M. from a city a thousand miles away. We would spend about a half hour on the wire, she crying out for help from the curse of chronic alcoholism and I trying to help her hear the Shepherd's voice. What the future brought to her I do not know. She was referred to a pastor in her city. Maybe in God's good time this lost sheep would be in the fold. Maybe not.

FORSAKEN?—NEVER!

"He heals the brokenhearted and binds up their wounds" (Psalm 147:3).

The ways of life are strange and hard. Most people battle them and manage to overcome with the aid and encouragement of good friends and the love of families. But some people have no close friends or family. Yet they survive because their best Friend, the Good Shepherd, keeps his promise to be with them always.

This is the lot of many chronic sufferers who have to live in an institution for ten, twenty, thirty years and more. They are forgotten and all alone in this big, bad world.

Emma was one of the unfortunates to be born with mental health issues. In spite of all then-known treatments for her condition, there was no help. Life became a static existence leading to a robot-like day-to-day routine among hundreds of others in similar circumstances. In more than twenty years she had had no visitor, except the pastor who toured the wards of the hospital.

Fortunately, she had been taught the essentials of God's truths and was able to draw much solace from the divine promises. But when one is all alone in the world and in the drab little rooms of a large mental health hospital, it must be doubly difficult to retain a hope for eventual relief from your griefs. Our Emma, however, persisted. She never missed a Sunday chapel service or a Communion opportunity, and that was the way the Holy Spirit kept her faith and hope alive and healthy.

When Emma became critically ill, a desperate attempt was made by the hospital's social service department to find some relative who might bring a little joy into this sad life that was soon to end. (Everyone who knew Emma was drawn to her in compassion because of her quiet, cooperative, and kind nature.)

Surprise! The old records in her file indicated that a grandniece upstate had at one time inquired about Emma's welfare. Though the address was from long ago, it still proved to be the residence of this distant relative. And when she was notified of Emma's condition, she immediately made the trip to Milwaukee and visited her great-aunt. What happiness there was for both! It was wonderful to behold. Emma was so pleased and her newly-found relative also, especially when they learned that they had a common bond of faith in the Lord Jesus. For the few weeks that remained of the patient's life, this grand-niece made a weekly and sometimes a twice-weekly trip to see Emma. And when Emma died, in her sixties, she was lovingly cared for in the arrangements for the burial.

A kind local mortician, a fellow-believer, treated this case of poverty and dependency as he would have dealt with a very profitable burial of any well-to-do client. He provided the casket and all necessary services at no cost to the one relative who remained.

What I will never forget about this lonely sheep of the flock is the scene at the funeral home the night before the burial. Emma had two callers: the niece and I. In the largest chapel of this home there were hundreds of people paying their respects to a prominent businessman of the area. The room overflowed with floral tributes. The casket was of bronze and all the appointments lavish. What a contrast! Wealth and poverty; thousands of friends and almost none; recognition by many and total anonymity!

Yet, the mortician was absolutely correct when he said to me, "Look at the difference between these two. But in heaven they are alike, the one a king and the other a queen before Jesus' throne. I'm glad we have pastors who go to any kind of people to show them the way to heaven."

How true! The Good Shepherd, through his undershepherds, kept close watch over both these souls, that neither might forfeit the prized crown.

FROM DEATH TO LIFE

Drug abuse is a problem that is maiming emotional stability in men, women, and even children. Drugs, of course, are a gift of God when used properly with professional advice. But they can produce devilish results and bring death of body and soul to those who abuse them.

In the emergency or trauma rooms of a large general hospital, there is a steady, daily stream of victims of accidents, shootings, and slashings, in addition to the more usual cases of physical illnesses. Statistics would verify the contention that many of the "accidents" are directly related to drug abuse.

Very early one morning, I was called to the intensive care unit to minister to a youth still in his twenties. He was from an eastern state and had come to our city with his girlfriend to visit her sister. It seems there had been serious disagreements in the young man's family over his use of "grass" and other mood-elevating drugs, and he was estranged from his parents. While on a "high," this trip was concocted as a lark.

The girlfriend's sister was another youthful wanderer who had come here and had "married" a casual acquaintance met at a "pot party." The visitors from Boston stayed in the sister's small apartment in one of the less desirable areas of the city. The day they arrived they were told by the "husband" that his "wife" was in a hospital awaiting the arrival of her first child. And when information came that the baby was born, he disappeared for several hours and did not return to the apartment until about 3:00 A. M., crazed by drugs and completely out of his mind. He imagined that his visitors were dangerous intruders and therefore grabbed a kitchen knife and began to slash away at them.

The youth from the east, sleeping on the floor in his sleeping bag, awoke suddenly when he felt deep pain and discovered blood flowing over his cheeks. As he looked up, he saw the man standing over him and stabbing away with the knife, until everything seemed to be red with blood. He became hysterical, but somehow managed to crawl to the hallway and cry for help. Someone heard him and called the police and an ambulance.

Later at the hospital the surgical team counted over 100 wounds, some superficial and some very deadly, near the heart. As one surgeon said: "When we got one wound patched, a half-dozen others were still spurting. As fast as we transfused blood into that body it kept running out!" But finally the four-hour rescue attempt was over and Ralph was moved to the recovery room.

When I first saw him there, he was in a state of shock. There would be a few waking moments, then a lapsing back into unconsciousness. In those waking moments I got close to his ear and repeated words of the Bible: "All we like sheep have gone astray . . . There is none that doeth good and sinneth not . . . Come now, let us reason together. Though your sins be as scarlet, they shall be white as snow." As he started to revive more completely, it was easy to direct him to his only Helper, the Shepherd Jesus. He knew the Lord. He had been confirmed as a youth in the Lutheran Church, but in a situation like this and with spiritual sensitivity high because death was so near, it called for repetition of those words that assure us of God's grace always being greater than our sins.

Over the weeks of recuperation that followed, quite a friendship was formed between us, and the young man poured out his heart to me. He told about his rebellion against his parents—how the reminder hurt now! He spoke of his foolish runaway attempt in coming to Milwaukee—how conscience shamed him now! He hadn't learned to appreciate his parents' insistence on good behavior and the right kind of friends and strict self-discipline. He thought he had found freedom, but now saw it as it was: self-imposed slavery. He knew he had been all wrong in following the desires of the flesh, and he meekly pleaded for forgiveness at the throne of mercy. When his parents were notified, they immediately flew to visit him. Ralph wanted me there when they arrived, and I was happy to oblige,

What a tearful reunion we witnessed! But if tears can be called bitter or sweet, these were all sweet. They were tears of thankfulness to a Shepherd who had guarded his sheep in danger and led it out of peril. Both parents and wayward son were grateful to him who "doeth all things well", even though the "things" included this horrible happening.

In a few more weeks Ralph was well enough to return to his home. He needed no more tranquilizers to make him tranquil and no more "uppers" to produce a feeling of euphoria. He had found a remedy for the ups and downs in life in him who can fill any heart and mind with perfect peace.

CONSTANT CONSOLATION

At some point in life, and perhaps more often than we care to remember, all of us live in a state of confusion. That's not a new psychological discovery. The reality of it is as old as man. David once said: "I have strayed like a lost sheep" (Psalm 119:176). Such a temporary state of confusion can do much harm before it is dispelled by the power of the Word.

A highly respected employee came to work one morning and was greeted by the news that she had been promoted to a very responsible and exacting position in her department. It was a time of elation, because it reflected the confidence the employer had in Clara. Being a humble Christian, Clara, with other serious thoughts in her mind at the time, was overwhelmed by the new turn of events which demanded an immediate decision.

What a spot for Satan to enter in! He helps to multiply the pressures and then tempts to evil. That's what he did to Clara. Momentarily stunned and confused, she tried to throw all the problems out of the window by ending them once and for all—in death! She ingested a powerful chemical by mouth.

She was immediately rushed to the intensive care unit, where every conceivable treatment was used to spare her life. The Shepherd too was not far afield, but watched the frantic doctoring and directed the hands of those who were trying to help Clara. And in his good time he approached the bedside in the person of one of his undershepherds. His voice was assuring through the Word.

On regaining consciousness this trembling sheep, aware of her critical self-imposed condition, wept tears. They were not tears of disappointment, but tears of gratitude at the assurance of divine forgiveness for the rash act.

Clara's confinement was long and often painful. There were numerous surgeries to help undo the damage done by the chemical. In all that time and through all the procedures there was never a complaint from this long-suffering sheep. In fact, she was a model to others in patience and endurance. It was a distinct privilege to have a part in reinforcing her spiritual needs.

From shadows to sunshine, from darkness to light—that might well be the theme of Clara's life today. It is. She proves it every day in her devotion to the Lord who has redeemed her.

LONG-TERM PATIENTS

Today, much emphasis is placed on the use of halfway houses as rehabilitation centers for those who will never be mentally well, but who at the same time can care for themselves in most ways. Many patients also are placed into nursing homes.

What a privilege it is for us to conduct services for them and keep them close to their Shepherd. Some of these patients have been with us for twenty-five to thirty years and are regular communicants. They also are sheep of his pasture and need to be fed regularly by the Word.

We have served one family of four sisters for longer than we care to remember. One of them died after lobectomy surgery; another passed away of natural causes. The two remaining have but one hope—that the Lord will soon relieve them of all the miseries of a sinful world and take them home for the grand reunion.

Others continue to walk difficult paths, aware of and enduring their personal eccentricities, while at the same time hating their own involuntary words and actions. No wonder they love their church service and their opportunities for the sacrament. For many, this has become the one and all of life—hearing the voice of the Good Shepherd, Jesus Christ.

HOW STRANGE ARE GOD'S WAYS!

Many unfortunate sufferers find ways to express their gratitude for the love of God. We read this in the things they do and say in their desire to tell us what is in their head.

When she first came to the hospital, Jane was completely out of contact with reality. She remained for a long time in a shell in her own little world. But after much therapy, she started to take interest in things around her, including, especially, the chapel where she often attended services. When she was permitted certain freedoms, you could often find her sitting on the floor before the chapel doors. She would spend hours there drawing pictures on burlap with crayons, and almost always the pictures were religious in nature. All one had to do was to give her a picture of postcard size and she would duplicate it in much larger dimensions on her canvas.

To this day, the lobby before the chapel is decorated with beautiful scenes she has produced, all of them biblical and accurately depicted. And out in the large ward corridors, dozens and dozens of her works of secular art are displayed as a testimony to her outstanding ability. Up in the superintendent's office there hangs a canvas done by her, about eight feet by twelve feet in size, showing the familiar picture of a doctor sitting at the side of a sick child's bed. And in my home hallway I have her three by four-foot crayon drawing of a retriever dog coming up out of the water with a duck in its mouth. Beautiful work she did. It made her happy.

She is today at a halfway house, aging rapidly and having lost her interest in what now would be a difficult task for her. One thing we hope she will never lose—the ability and desire to hear her Shepherd's voice saying, "Come unto me."

Original poem by a patient in a psychiatric hospital ward:

> *TRUTH and LOVE*
>
> *All mortals who in truth adhere,*
> *Shall dwell in love and know no fear. For love and truth go hand in hand.*
> *This JESUS taught, so understand. That all who crave a life of love,*
> *Must turn their thought to God above.*
>
> *For God doth ever dwell in him,*
> *Who cleans his mind from mortal sin. And he in love shall take their hand,*
> *And lead them to the promised land. Where hate and malice are unknown,*
> *For God sits there upon his throne.*
>
> *But they who fail to live in truth,*
> *Shall lose all honor and their youth. And live in turmoil and in pain,*
> *Until they bow their heads in shame. And turn again to God above,*
> *And seek his aid with TRUTH and LOVE.*
>
> *E. Mavis*

REBELLIOUS AND DISCIPLINED SHEEP

In several passages the Bible speaks of "sheep going astray." It seems to be a natural habit of sheep to wander off and get themselves into situations of fear and danger. They may also be stolen by false shepherds in their wanderings and find themselves in captivity.

So it is with people. Bad habits, plain stupidity, covetousness, and greed, all these are contributing factors to their delinquency. And when they become angry with themselves and with society, they strike back in rebellion against "the system." If their rebellious habit is not checked and their offenses against others are grave enough, they need to be corrected forcibly. They have to spend time in jail or prison.

For some, this is a blessing in disguise. They learn to listen closely for the Shepherd's voice; they learn to long for pardon and peace. Then when the gospel is preached behind prison walls, the Holy Spirit uses it to restore the potentially lost sinner to sonship in the kingdom.

PRISON WITNESS

Johnny was the only son of well-to-do farmers. By the time he was fifteen years old, his parents had bought a farm in his name and established a sizable bank account for him.

They gave him all the money he wanted to use and let him know by word and deed that nothing was too good for him. It was a perfect pattern for teaching the child to worship at the shrine of materialism and personal satisfactions at any cost.

The seeds that had been sown sprouted and flowered. But what horrible fruit they produced! There came the evening when, for some reason, the parents denied Johnny the use of the farm truck to visit some neighbor boys. He pouted, he became angrier by the minute, and finally he was furious enough to be uncontrollable. He ran to his upstairs room, got his shotgun, ran back down to the kitchen and shot his mother through the head. She died almost instantly. The father, who was also in the kitchen, would have suffered a similar fate. But Johnny's foot slipped, the aim was off target, and the shot missed its mark. The father fled to the barn for protection.

Since this was a capital crime demanding a penalty of imprisonment in a maximum security prison, the lad at fifteen was taken to the State Penitentiary, where I met the young murderer among a large number of criminals of every description. Some were calloused and hardened repeaters. Most of them were cold and indifferent to the real meaning of life, astray from their best and most helpful Friend, the Shepherd Jesus.

When I received his admission card and saw that he was listed as a Lutheran, I had him brought into the office for an interview. It was the only time through thirty years of prison mission work that I had ever met a boy of his tender age in prison as a murderer. He must be tough and cruel in nature, I thought. What could I possibly do to lead him correctly?

At our first meeting I could sense his feelings of isolation and loneliness, his fear of many of the men around him, and his feelings of hopelessness for the future. Believe me, my heart was soft toward this frightened and trembling sheep. And as we talked, I had to add to his discomfort by reminding him sternly of his offense against God and the even worse penalty he would have to face before God's perfect court of justice—hell! He hadn't had much religious training at all, just a casual knowledge of church, gained from attending relatives' weddings or funerals. And so, all the fundamentals of truth were new and impressive. He was specially puzzled by the Bible's promise of forgiveness for all sin through the life and death of the "Shepherd of Israel."

Johnny readily accepted our invitation to join the class that was studying the Bible and Catechism, and his spiritual growth from month to month stood out in the questions he asked and the occasional comments he made. He was a bright boy and read every bit of religious material I could supply for him, zeroing in on those precious promises of pardon.

In good time, the Spirit let the voice of the Good Shepherd come through loud and clear and, after witnessing the confirmation of one class, he requested that he be included in the next. Naturally, his wish was granted, and about a year later another found sheep was returned to the flock. He attended all our chapel services and partook of the Lord's body and blood at every opportunity.

His spiritual beauty wasn't just skin deep. His devotion to the Lord made him want to be a witness to Christ in the whole prison compound. So he began a study of music with the intent of becoming chapel organist someday. He studied and practiced for many months; almost all his free time was used in this way. His persistence paid off. He could play the hymns very well. A goal had been reached when he was given permission to serve our "congregation" of about 170 attendees. He retained that position for six years.

Time moves swiftly when one is occupied with doing things that please you in service to others, mainly to God. So Johnny's time was served. And though it did not seem possible, the fifteen years he spent with us came to an end. Because of his good record, he was released after serving the minimum time demanded by law. Johnny had to leave the relative shelter and security of prison life.

Unfortunately, we did not have the facilities for close follow-up on released prisoners, and so we had to trust that somehow, the Shepherd would keep his sheep within range of his voice. We established contact with a pastor on the outside and plunged back into the large pool of opportunities that always faced us wherever doors were open to us.

It is always a pleasure and satisfaction to meet a released prisoner years after his imprisonment and hear him tell that he is a member of such and such church, still joined to the flock. It was a special joy to meet Johnny about ten years later in one of our churches at a worship service. He had married a good Christian wife and was the proud father of two little boys. Sitting behind this family in a church we were visiting one evening, we couldn't help noticing the rapt interest of the boys in everything that was going on. One of the boys had his eyes glued to the pastor as he officiated at the altar or in the pulpit. At the end of the service, those little eyes followed the pastor down the center aisle to the narthex of the church, where he was greeting parishioners. There was a smile on the boy's face, and when his chance came to shake hands with the pastor, the eyes literally glistened. It was obvious that he was a very happy lad.

In the narthex a few minutes later, I approached my former confirmand and chatted with him about past events, expressing my happiness at seeing him. While we were talking about how good God had been to him in his new life, the little boy tugged on his father's coat, pointed at me and asked, "Dad, is that a pastor?" Johnny introduced us, and the lad said with unmistakable determination, "Someday I'm going to be a pastor too!"

We might title this sheep's story: "From tragedy to triumph." For the powerful call of the Shepherd's voice had accomplished its purpose in Johnny's life and was continuing to be a guiding light for him and his family.

Maybe too the little boy's wish will come true.

THROUGH TRIBULATION TO HEAVEN

"We must go through many hardships to enter the kingdom of God" (Acts 14:22). How often haven't we heard those words? But their real meaning is not impressed on us until we ourselves are being tried in the fires of purification, or until someone we know intimately is made to pass from one crisis to another until peace is reestablished in his or her soul.

John Jay was one who was severely tried until he met the Good Shepherd Jesus and learned to listen to his voice.

John was born and raised in an isolated rural area of the state, far removed from the advantages of normal educational facilities. Nor was there any church within many miles of his home. He was a boy easily taught, but his skills developed almost exclusively in the practice of farming and later he became a "herdsman," a tender of cattle.

In his mid-twenties, he married and proved to be a dependable and faithful husband to his young wife. He loved her about as much as you can love anyone who joins you daily in hard work to make a living and see the fulfillment of mutual dreams.

After a number of years of happy marriage, John Jay came home one day from his weekly shopping trip to a neighboring town. Up the driveway he noticed a strange truck, and when he entered the kitchen he heard his wife's screams for help. In the bedroom, a man was attacking and assaulting his wife! Naturally, John rushed in to defend her from harm. And in doing this according to his natural instincts, he beat the attacker unmercifully into unconsciousness and almost to death.

Applied to such cases, the law is sometimes strangely misapplied. John soon learned that. He was accused of criminal assault against the intruder, tried in court, and sent to prison for five years! He was confused and understandably angry and helpless. His adjustment to prison life was complicated more than usual because he was worrying about his wife and her welfare back home. "There must be more to life than this," was his growing conviction. Without his knowing it, his distasteful experiences were opening a door for the Good Shepherd.

A fellow inmate, noticing John Jay's discomfort and misery, invited him to attend the chapel services one Sunday morning. He followed his friend and came. This was all so new to John: grown men singing hymns, listening to a preacher read and preach from the Bible, and bowing their heads and folding their hands in prayer.

The Bible was a book he knew by name, but he had never read in it. Consequently, he had no way of knowing its purpose or possible effect on his thinking and behavior, or its direction to a life much more important and perfect than the years we live on earth. Yet John was willing to learn, and so he continued to attend chapel, while all along the Holy Spirit was leading him to the gate of the sheepfold.

After several months, John Jay felt bold enough to ask for an interview. He frankly told the story of his life and asked for permission to attend the class that was digging deeper into God's truth in special sessions every time the pastor made his visits to the prison.

Then came the day, a long time later, when the course was completed. The men were quizzed as to their understanding of law and gospel and other basics in the Christian faith and were then invited to participate in the privileges and responsibilities of church membership. Not all accepted, but John Jay was one of several who sincerely desired to follow through and "join the church." I shall never forget that day when, in the presence of a "congregation" of about twenty eligible communicants, John made his confession of faith, was baptized and confirmed, and for the first time in his life received the body and blood of our Lord in Holy Communion.

I shall never forget the day because, as we confessed our sins and the absolution from guilt was pronounced in the service, John instinctively knelt before his chair and unashamedly shed tears of mingled sorrow and joy at the thought of God's love for him, a wandering and undeserving sinner. Now he knew the sweet mystery of life, which had eluded him for so many years. He became a daily reader of Scriptures and never failed to attend the services and the monthly Communion.

About three years later he became seriously ill. At a state hospital he was put through many tests and finally told that cancer cells had invaded his body and that the outlook was anything but promising. For months he spent much time on a bed of pain, but he never became hopelessly discouraged. He fastened his eyes heavenward and prayed for release into the heavenly sheepfold.

Some friends brought his case to the attention of the governor's pardon counsel toward year's end. And when the medics predicted that this patient would not live out the year, the governor magnanimously signed a pardon for John and had it presented to him on Christmas Eve. The pardon, of course, indicated that this lawbreaker had paid his debt to society in full and was once again a free man. The public press made much of this gracious act, using it as an example of the spirit of Christmas. It was heart warming to read the story in the papers on the eve of Christmas, as we were getting ready for the children's service that would reecho the good news: "Unto YOU is born a Savior." The air seemed crisper, the snow whiter. All was well with the world of God's sheep!

The doctors were right. John Jay died a few days later and, in spirit, joined the angel choirs as they repeated, "Glory to God in the highest." He was relieved of all earthly troubles. So often, still, I think about John and what the power of God's Word did for him. And the thought just will not die: If we might be able to talk to the man today and ask him which pardon means more to him, the one signed by the governor or the one signed by Jesus' blood, I'm sure what the answer would be. It would be an unmistakable testimony to God's goodness in sending the Shepherd to seek the lost sheep, fold them in his powerful arms, care for them even in the days of tribulation, and finally lead them to eternal glory.

KNOWLEDGE WITHOUT WISDOM

Eddie graduated from high school with honors. He was exceptionally intelligent and well-trained in many fields of learning. He was happy to grasp every opportunity offered him in America after his parents had brought him here from Europe. A successful future in life was almost guaranteed.

Eddie's parents were industrious people, and they saw in our country great opportunities that they had never dreamed about in their homeland: opportunities for freedoms of every kind and security by hard and honest labor. As Eddie and his brother grew into manhood they enjoyed learning and earning. They looked ahead to the days when they would have to deny themselves nothing.

And then tragedy entered Eddie's life. He fell in love with one of his schoolmates and intended to marry her as soon as he had saved enough to set up his own home. During the courtship his girlfriend became pregnant, and Eddie was frantic because his parents had set a high code of personal honor and decency for the family. Exposure of his indiscretion and sin would mean deep trouble for both families involved in the situation.

The girl confided in her younger sister who began to taunt Eddie and make threats to tell the parents the sad story. The consequences could be disastrous! In a flash Eddie lost his power of reason and murdered the sister by shooting her. Then, tying a building block to her body, he dropped it into a deep harbor at the lake front. So he hoped to prevent discovery of the body and cover his criminal act.

Accidentally, the police discovered the body a few days after, as they were dragging the harbor in search of a reported suicide. It was identified by relatives, and an intense investigation was started. Piece by piece, the picture was put together and the finger of guilt pointed to Eddie, who in the meantime, had left the city with his new bride after a hasty marriage ceremony. The two were quickly tracked down about three hundred miles from home. Eddie was arrested and charged and returned for trial in court. The charge was first degree murder! And that meant a life sentence in the penitentiary on conviction. To his credit, it must be said that Eddie did not try to evade the truth and excuse his horrible sin, in spite of the fact that he knew it would mean the end of all those great dreams for a happy life in America. All hopes were dashed on the rocks of rebellion against the law and against God.

I met the young man at the prison sometime later at the request of the warden. He was concerned that the blasé attitude of this intelligent youth indicated a false sense of self-understanding that could lead to serious mental problems later on. I recall the warden saying: "I feel that soon he may be 'blowing his top' unless we can bring him to a solid sense of reality."

Working with Eddie became a real pleasure, not because of his natural attitude, but because of his willingness to accept help and love. Here was a lost sheep filled with trembling and feelings of insecurity that were being buried under a blasé demeanor. Of the many fine things Eddie's parents had provided for him, there was a most needful element lacking, and that was the anchor of religion. Because of some unhappy religious experiences the family had had overseas, the young man knew little of God, of sin, and of pardon and restoration.

Eagerly he absorbed the many newly-found truths of the Scriptures in his private study of the Bible and in our group classes. When we studied the sacrament of baptism, for instance, he waited after the class one day to inquire about how he could shoulder his responsibility to his new daughter by bringing her to the Good Shepherd. At his request we arranged the baptism in our home with the mother being a willing participant, though she was of a very strict "other religion."

But the Shepherd had not finished his work among the members of this family. I supplied a Catechism for Eddie's parents and their son's family, now living with them, so that they might understand what was bringing their loved one his deepest satisfaction in those awful days behind prison walls. This led to a whole chain of events that brought joy to the angels in heaven.

Eddie's wife studied the Catechism, spoke about it with her family, was instructed by a local pastor and confirmed. Her trust in the gospel of God's promises infected others, so that before long they followed her example and entered the fold with her to live in that "peace which by far surpasses all human understanding."

After more than twelve years, Eddie was paroled from prison with an excellent record. The once straying and lost sheep were reunited to enjoy the gentle care and right direction of the Shepherd, who leads his own to eternal joys.

STRESSED TO THE BREAKING POINT

Not only young and middle-aged men and women are sent to prison for crimes, but also aged folk who are guilty of serious crimes. And then, of course, there are those who have grown old while serving their sentences imposed in earlier years.

Woodrow had been a wanderer in his early years. He had little respect for formal schooling. He preferred to learn by seeing and doing. His self-adopted lifestyle explains his many meanderings in our country and abroad.

In later years he settled down and decided to be a meat cutter. He was good at his work and soon acquired ownership of a market which grew into a thriving and lucrative business. His marriage to a good woman and the raising and educating of a family marked him as a successful man. His reputation was above reproach.

Close as the family members were, they never felt that they knew him very well; there seemed to be so much that he kept all to himself.

After many years of wedded contentment, his wife became ill with a painful and crippling malady. Eventually all her waking hours were spent in a wheelchair. The children were gone and busy rearing their own families. Contact was minimal. So every day before opening the shop Woodrow would help his wife out of bed, dress and groom her, help her into her wheelchair, feed her, and then set her at a table. The door between the shop and living quarters was kept open so that he could keep watch over her and respond to her signal for help. He prepared her meals and at day's end and helped her to bed. Many times each day he would spend a moment or two with her to buoy up her spirit. But for a man of his particular nature, this deadly routine drained him emotionally and made him function almost like a robot. His wanderlust returned to him.

He developed a strong habit of feeling sorry for himself, and his pride prevented him from asking others for help. Soon every trip into the kitchen was a temptation to sip a little brandy or wine, so that by the end of the day he scarcely knew what he was doing. On one weekend, while he was thoroughly intoxicated, the devilish thought came to rid himself of the heavy burden by doing away with his wife. A cleaver, a knife, and soon the body were incinerated in the furnace! Is something so revolting really possible? Later, Woodrow himself would tell you that unbelievable things can happen when you forget God and let the devil rule over your thoughts and actions.

Woodrow's crime could not remain concealed for long. Suspicion was aroused when the wife was no longer seen at her customary place. Friends were evaded when they called. A tip to the police resulted in a thorough investigation, and an unhappy, guilty man confessed what he had done. The shock of it all led to deep shame and disgrace, and when the judge pronounced a life sentence for the crime, life suddenly appeared to have ended for Woodrow.

I met him during his first weeks of confinement in prison. He was a grandfatherly, docile man easy to talk with. He was completely sorry for what he had done, but not totally aware of the seriousness and consequences of his crime of murder. Now in the declining years of his life—in the seventies—he resigned himself to slow death and a life of grieving.

After numerous visits he became attracted to our chapel services and a bit later asked to join the instruction class. The Bible and Catechism were not entirely strange to him, but over the years he forgot more than he retained. And so he appreciated going over the basics and had a special interest in a review of the Second Article of the Creed which told the story of God's love for the sinner through the Savior Jesus.

God forgives? Yes. God forgives ALL sins? Yes. God can forgive murder? Yes, he can and he does if the murderer is led to lay his sin and guilt at the foot of Jesus' cross. That cross, after all, was the payment in full for every man's transgressions of whatever kind and quantity.

As unbelievable as his crime now was to Woodrow, so unbelievable was the depth of God's love for the fallen. It was unbelievable until the Holy Spirit enlightened this unhappy man and tended the weak plant of faith in his heart. He dared believe; he did believe with all his heart that his Shepherd loved him and had died for him!

More than a year later Woodrow was ready to make his vows to the Triune God. It was a bright day in his life when he was confirmed and received the sacrament of pardon. From then on, he seldom missed a worship service or any opportunity to be reassured at the Lord's Table. Our many private conversations reaffirmed his sincerity and his desire to give his life to the Lord for all eternity.

As an older man he was not made to work daily as were the younger prisoners. Consequently he spent much of his time making articles of jewelry, making greeting cards (all with religious sentiments), and doing much reading in the Bible and devotional literature. Woodrow became an example to many in his cell block and a friend to hundreds in the prison compound.

When the minimum requirements of his sentence were met, after quite a few years, he was released on parole. The family had no room for him at this late hour in life, and he was sent to a public home for dependent elderly people. As soon as he arrived at his new home he notified me of his whereabouts, and we kept up the regular contact with spiritual ministration for a number of years. What an encouragement these visits were for me in a lonely ministry! To hear this aged "ex-con" sing the praises of a marvelous Father in heaven who had shepherded him through strange ways to make life meaningful and filled with hope—this was a strengthening tonic in a ministry that daily dealt in heartaches!

Today Woodrow lives out his remaining days in another institution. He is no longer of agile mind. Yet, like Simeon of old, he waits for the joy of seeing his Savior face to face. The Shepherd knows where he is; no one shall ever pluck him out of his hand.

HARDENED TO SOFTNESS

In prison one meets all sorts of people. Some are constantly surly and sullen; others are covetous and cruel; some are brazen and bullish in their attitude toward other people. When one approaches them in the role of pastor or chaplain, he can almost feel the deadliness of Satan's success with them.

But we dare never underestimate the greater power of God's Word. Patience in applying truth can bring happy rewards. This was illustrated in the case of a repeater who was sent back to prison many times on burglary and armed robbery charges. He never seemed to learn the lesson that crime does not pay but exacts heavy tribute.

At various times he was in our classes, probably just out of curiosity or for the break from humdrum work and the routine of prison living. He was always welcomed and made to feel that God was interested in his fragmented life.

Several years had passed when one day he surprised me with his request for confirmation and Communion. He was taken into the class and many months later baptized, confirmed, and communed. There was an obvious transformation in his life that was noticed by many. In fact, a number of other prisoners were moved to join future classes by their contact with this "new man."

On his release from confinement, I lost track of him because he had left no forwarding address at which we might reach him. But about a year later, there was an urgent long-distance phone call from him in which he asked me to call on his mother. She lived in our city, and we were happy to comply. In a ramshackle residence we found a woman of about sixty years, dying of cancer.

She had had no church contacts, knew exceptionally little about God, and was afraid to die. When he learned of her fear and despair, her son, our confirmand, was convinced that she must hear what God had to offer in his Word. (Unknown to me, he had become a member of a church upstate and was active in helping the youth of the congregation in various programs.)

Through many hardships and disappointing experiences in life, the mother's heart had been cultivated into fertile soil for the seeds of truth. Almost daily in her final months of life on earth, I was at her bedside instructing, convicting, comforting, and encouraging her to grasp God's promises in faith. The seeds brought their fruit. She believed simply, humbly, but also powerfully. To the joy of people and angels she was relieved of all suffering and taken to her heavenly home.

Quite some time passed, and then again there was a phone call from the son. Would I please call on the father of this family? He was an emergency admission to the Medical Complex after suffering a damaging heart attack. Condition: "Critical, and most likely terminal."

The son had warned me that this would not be an easy case, since the father was a hardened, crude, and salty individual, who gave no quarter to anyone. His evaluation was an understatement. Yet I reminded the son, and myself, that with God all things are possible. He can turn the most hardened sinner into a saint. The miracle can happen through his Word.

The reception at my first visit was anything but encouraging, and I felt ill at ease. After several visits, however, the rebellion against God began to ease, and the man was ready to listen to what God might say to him. With his wife and son as examples of unworthy sinners being led to peace with God, his interest grew into acceptance, hoping, and believing. His days were numbered. He knew it. And in the few days that remained, he looked forward daily to hearing: "My son be of good cheer; thy sins are forgiven thee." He died peacefully in the Lord.

I often think of this family and of what might have happened or not happened to it if an unruly son had not found the Shepherding Christ while he was in prison. "I was in prison and you came to visit me," Jesus said. How many more rebellious sheep will meet their greatest joy behind walls of shame and disgrace?

Would we ever deny them the opportunity?

DEDICATION IN RESTORATION

"I am an inmate at the state prison," wrote the middle-aged man from a small interrelated rural community, "and I have had the pleasure of hearing you preach in the chapel three times so far. I have enjoyed your sermons very much. They lift me up out of the depths of sin, shame, and humiliation. The first sermon I heard you preach was taken from Isaiah 1:18. I shall never forget the text, 'Come now, let us reason together,' says the LORD. 'Though your sins are like scarlet, they shall be as white as snow; though they are red as crimson, they shall be like wool.' When next you come to the prison I would like to confess my sins to you. I was raised in a Christian home and went to Sunday school and church and was also baptized. But for some reason or other, I let Jesus out of my life and fell into the path of sin which leads to the destruction of the mind, body, and soul. But thank God! It is not too late for me to repent and confess my sins and be saved by the grace of Jesus Christ our Lord. I want to be a Christian man and have a Christian home. I want to bring up my family that way."

That was the first part of a letter I received a few days after one of our chapel services at the prison. The remainder spelled out, in detail, the man's family circumstances and the "back-sliding" that ended in prison on a shameful admitted charge of gross immoral conduct. The offense was so grievous in the community that the sentencing judge said publicly: "We never want to see you in this town again." And those words haunted and taunted Chris many, many times during long and sleepless nights in his cell.

In those solitary hours he kept thinking: "If my relatives and friends at home can be so incensed at what I've done (and they have a perfect right to feel as they do), what God must think of my sinful act?" Day by day the self-condemnation grew until he was in a state of near despair.

One Sunday morning, when chapel call rang through the tiers of cells, some inner voice urged him to join the line forming for the march to chapel. He went. And he came again a second time, and a third. That third Sunday afternoon he sat down to write the letter quoted above. He had heard the voice of the Good Shepherd inviting him to peace for his troubled soul.

A long and beautiful shepherding relationship followed. He never missed a class or a service. He read his Bible every day and prayed a lot. "I have confessed my sins to God, and I am sure he has forgiven me for Jesus' sake," he said. He often repeated the words of St. John: "If we claim to be without sin, we deceive ourselves and the truth is not in us. If we confess our sins, he is faithful and just and will forgive us our sins and purify us from all unrighteousness." (1 John 1:8, 9).

After this lost sheep had been found and helped back to the fold, he was so strong in his reliance on God's help and goodness that he even did "the hard things of rehabilitation." On release from prison he returned to the old home town, bravely faced the snubs of townsmen and church people until finally all were convinced of his sincerity and "rebirth." It wasn't easy, and it took a long time. When the going was unusually tough, he would write for reassurance and encouragement in the hope that was so strong while he was in confinement. He prayed that it might continue to support him until life's end.

NATURAL MAN

In ministering to prisoners for thirty years, one Scripture truth has become imbedded in my mind. It is that natural man is an enemy of God and opposed to every expression of his will and way. "There is no one who does good, not even one." "We all, like sheep, have gone astray, each of us has turned to his own way."

The modern doctrine that tells us that all are born good and in innocence is a devilish falsehood. To support their false doctrine, some will blame environment and negative circumstances for evidences of evil and crime in people. But this is simply closing our eyes to reality. The following item from a recent newspaper release ought to teach all a solemn lesson.

12-YEAR-OLD GETS 25 YEARS FOR MURDER

Miami, Fla. - AP - A 12-year-old boy, known as "Little Shorty" to his friends in sixth grade, has been sentenced to 25 years in prison for murder, robbery, and burglary. He will be eligible for parole after one year.

Erwin H - pleaded no contest to second degree murder. He was the youngest of five youths charged with fatally beating an 85-year-old man while burglarizing his home in February.

A 13-year-old codefendant, Eve P., was sentenced to 114 years in prison. Prosecutors charged that she was the leader in the murder of Ralph G., who died of a crushed skull more than a month after the Feb. 7 beating.

How fortunate and blessed are those who are born into Christian homes and learn to heed the way of God's righteousness.

A SCARY SUNDAY NIGHT

It will happen that sheep, fairly new to the fold, have to grow in their confidence of the Shepherd's leadership. Meanwhile, they may often tremble, be scared, and in panic easily do things for which they are sorry later.

Tim was somewhat shiftless in his early years. Weak family influences were of no help in the confusing processes of growing up. But after high school years and a period of gainful employment, he seemed to become more stable and responsible. Yet when he married a good Christian girl a few years later, the new responsibilities of being a husband and provider began to overpower him. Soon there were pressing financial obligations; his creditors were hounding him; and he needed to find extra sources of cash supply.

It was an easy step from stealing to burglary and then to armed robbery, after listening to the optimistic advice of the wrong kind of friends. But it was also an easy step to growing conflicts with the law. Justice must be tempered with mercy, of course, but mercy must never be devoid of sound reasoning. Tim felt the sting of undue leniency in criminal courts when, after several sentences of probation, he was sent to prison for a period of several years.

Here his confusion multiplied and his restlessness was almost beyond control. Yet he followed orders and performed his duties, had a good behavior record, and was soon placed on an honor farm outside the prison walls. It raised his hopes for an early release.

A letter from his young wife, informing him that their awaited baby would be born soon, upset him. Emotionally unstable as he was, this news froze his reasoning powers. That night he escaped from the farm and made his way back home to be near his wife. He lived in hiding in her apartment. As he later said, he knew all along that his escape was wrong and that it would surely bring him an extension of his sentence, but under the stress of the moment he was not able to cope with these realities.

Imagine my surprise when late one Sunday evening our doorbell rang and a very frightened young woman stood on our step. Telling me who she was, she motioned to the shadows behind an evergreen, and quickly Tim was in our living room. I knew him from our contacts at the prison as a mild-mannered and friendly attendee at the chapel services, but now I faced a frightened and furtive youth capable of any kind of impulsive action.

The wife told me that Tim had often written to her. He had shared with her the hopes and dreams that were building up in him, as a result of the assurances that God is with his repentant children and will work out all things for their best. It was because of her understanding of Tim's growing reliance on God's truth that she was able to convince him to come to our home for counsel in this shaky situation.

At first as we talked, Tim was not willing to give himself up to the proper authorities. And I became uneasy in my role of temporarily harboring an escaped criminal. But finally he submitted, because he was convinced this was the thing God would want him to do.

I called an agent of the parole department at his home and was advised to give the couple a few dollars for a night's lodging away from their home, (it was being watched by state agents), and tell them to report to the parole officer first thing in the morning. This I did. But I feared that Tim might change his mind, and all of us would be involved in the consequences.

At about 8:05 the next morning, however, my fears were allayed when the officer called to say that my charge had arrived there. The officials would work out something to soften the blow of Tim's indiscretion.

Well, he was sent back to prison with an addition to his original sentence, behaved himself very well, had no demerit marks, and later was given an early release. To my knowledge, he has never again been in serious trouble.

He had learned to commit his way unto the Lord, and the Lord gave sustaining stamina to this troubled sheep. The Great Shepherd's tender care had rescued another rebellious sheep with discipline for his special needs. Probably never again will that voice be muted in the life of Tim and his closely-knit family.

THE WORD WILL NOT LET GO

When once a sheep begins to grasp the love, trust, and care of its shepherd, it is reluctant to leave that shepherd and his flock again. And when a Christian has tasted the Great Shepherd's love and learned to trust his ways, he does not ever again want to be separated from the flock.

I knew a man who spent many years of confinement in prison, years in which the Holy Spirit was enlightening his sin-darkened mind and calling him by the Word of God to a deeper knowledge of what life was all about. Then rather suddenly came his decision to join the flock of the Shepherd.

For many hours he sat in the classes, quietly absorbing the incredible fact that God doesn't want the death of any sinner, but that all should come to the knowledge of the truth and be saved. Before he could finish the course and be confirmed, prison officials felt that he was ready for a transfer to a state camp where he would be conditioned for a "life on the outside" after his full term was served.

Most men are happy for such an opportunity, but this man was not. In fact, he tried to have his transfer delayed to some future time. The reason, as he frankly stated it, was, "How could I complete my instruction in the north woods and become a member of the church?" It was only after he had been promised that we would have a pastor visit him there and continue to instruct him for full church membership, that he consented to the move.

A faithful pastor in the area drove about sixty miles roundtrip week after week until the man was ready to make his public confession of faith and dedication. Hank, as we called him, was a former agnostic and scoffer. On release from custody he became a member of the pastor's congregation.

In a subsequent letter to me that pastor wrote: "If you ever have any more men like Hank coming to this camp, please let me know. He has proved to be a real asset to our local church."

YOUNG, AGING, AND OLD SHEEP

The sheep of the flock are of all age groups. Some may be newborn infants, rejected by their parents, but claimed by the Shepherd. Such cases are brought to our attention, mainly by our "on-call" system at the Medical Complex.

A woman gives birth to a set of twins, but refuses even to look at them when the nurse brings them into her room for the first time. The nurse is a Christian, understandably concerned about baptism for the two tiny, helpless girls. So she calls the control center and summons a chaplain. He speaks with the mother and receives permission to baptize the children and to then refer the family to a neighborhood pastor. The Shepherd has kept watch, searched, and found!

Or a mother abandons a child born out of wedlock. Heartlessly she turns it over to the care of some public welfare system, and the child grows up in an institution, never knowing the love and comforts of a family home. During war years, we had over 800 such dependents in our one small area of the nation.

Ours was the privilege of teaching over 250 children the Word of a kind heavenly Father and conducting weekly church services for them. The Shepherd walked among these little sheep to protect them from the wolves' destruction.

NEVER ABANDONED BY GOD

We met tiny Pete in our Sunday school, conducted with the help of Seminary students and lay volunteers. He was a slow learner, but very sensitive and lovable. After a time, he attached himself to the "Lutheran priest" as his friend. There were no relatives he knew of. No one ever came to visit him. And our hearts were touched as we thought of his pitiful situation.

Abandoned as a baby and receiving loving care only vicariously from the staff of the Home, he grew up to lean heavily on any offer of kindness and interest that came his way. I believe that partly explains his unmistakable devotion to the many stories we told him about Jesus: the powerful and promising loving Friend of all children. His eyes seemed to grow larger and they glistened whenever he was reminded that Jesus had commanded his disciples to bring the young children to him, because they were a part of God's blessed family.

With many handicaps to overcome and not possessing a keen mind, Pete often was the recipient of pranks at the home. Some terrible things were said to him to scare him or force him to submit to the whims and demands of other children. But his tears could be dried easily by an arm around his shoulders or a friendly pat on the head. He was easily comforted, because he trusted he was "Jesus' boy."

In due time, Pete was in our instruction class preparing for confirmation. He was willing to remain in the class beyond the usual time so that he might memorize and master the truths that had become so dear to him. It was a happy day when he could stand before our altar and confess his faith with the class of confirmands. He was a fine young Christian, always in chapel services, always at the Lord's Table. This was the foundation for his friendliness, obedience, and contentment in his loneliness.

When children are in such a home for a long time (Pete was with us for fifteen years), the staff tries to find a family that will take them in and treat them as its own son or daughter. The day that a boy or girl is called into the superintendent's office and told that a home has been found is usually a very happy day. The children look with anticipation to meeting their new parents, having their own room and clothing, enjoying all the freedoms and advantages of family life. And they make the staff of the home happy by reacting accordingly.

But the day that Pete was called in to have his placement described was different. He showed no signs of exuberance, but only tolerance. The home was his only experience in living. He had grown accustomed to it as a pattern and feared any drastic change. He had learned much and had set his own certain ideals. They centered in his Savior Jesus.

So when the superintendent spoke with him, Pete asked: "Will these people help me get to church on Sundays?" Reassured that they had made that promise, Pete reacted like other happy youngsters anticipating a new life in new surroundings. He gladly consented to move to a rural farm, far removed from the only home he had ever known.

Six months later I received a scribbled letter, a letter I will always cherish, because it reminds me of the power of our God's holy Word in a person's life. Such a letter takes away all the remembrance of hard work, difficulties, and discouragements in the ministry. Pete described his new living conditions and experiences, and one could just feel the new zest in his being. He loved the animals he was allowed to tend on the farm. He gladly performed routine duties in doing chores and running errands. He was pleased with the kindnesses of everyone on the farm, especially of the hired hands who were so friendly. One of the hired men had become a "big brother" to Pete and helped him to save enough to buy a bicycle, his first very own earned possession!

The letter went on to tell how easy it now was to get to church without bothering anyone else. "With the bicycle it's no trouble at all. I jump on my bike, pedal the five miles to town to church, and then pedal home again." (How many of us would find this a pleasure and privilege?) And at the end of his letter Pete added: "Of course, when it rains it's not so good, because my bike has no mudguards on it."

A sheep found for the Lord's fold! What joy in heaven! What joy for us! We met Pete several times in later years, after he had returned to the city to find gainful employment. One of the first things he would mention was his present church connection and his joy in belonging to the Shepherd's family.

Pete, if you ever happen to read this story, you will certainly recognize yourself in it. Thank you for the encouragement and for the mighty lesson you have taught all of us by demonstrating the truth of the Word: "My Word will not return to me empty."

EMERGENCY BAPTISM

The little four-year-old looked even younger, as he lay on that big white hospital bed. He was so helpless and scared. He had been rushed to the hospital in an ambulance with flashing red lights and screaming sirens. He was gasping for breath as a result of some tracheal obstruction. It was determined swiftly that only surgery could save his life.

The chief surgeon on the case had to move quickly. Time was important. But being a committed Christian, he did not want to begin the surgery until he was assured that the boy had been baptized.

A ward official called the boy's home to inquire about his baptism. The sad answer was that the parents had not had time or opportunity to bring this lamb to the Shepherd for spiritual care! However, consent to baptize the boy was readily given when the father was told that a Lutheran pastor was available at the hospital to perform the sacrament.

So I was called, and within minutes stood at the boy's bed-side. Doctors and nurses were waiting to cart him off to the operating room. In the brief moments allowed me, I nervously tried to explain to the lad what happens to us when water is applied to our head in the name of the triune God. Faith is born, and in faith we are made his dear children, washed clean by Jesus' precious blood of all we have done wrong. What words I actually spoke in the brief time I had I do not remember exactly, but then the power is not in us, but in the Word of truth itself, as God has revealed it to us in Holy Scriptures.

The power of that Word was evident in this situation. When I asked him if he wanted to be Jesus' child, he nodded his head in assent. He was baptized as simply as possible and then, after a brief prayer asking the Good Shepherd to watch over this trembling lamb, the boy was whisked off to the operating room. My sleep was sporadic that night as I kept waking and thinking about the boy. Early the next morning I returned to his room to find him resting peacefully and breathing normally. His father was at the bedside. He lowered his head and folded his hands as we thanked God for preserving the son's life. Then the father followed me out of the room and in our conversation gave me the marvelous assurance that God had done his work well. The Word and sacrament had had its effect on the boy, as he himself testified to his father. For when they had conversed briefly that morning, and though it had been difficult to understand the youngster because of the tracheotomy tube in his throat, these are the happy words he heard from the boy: "Last night, after it was dark, a man from God came and made me a child of Jesus."

The Holy Spirit surely had enlightened that little mind through the Word spoken to him. He came to know and trust the love of the great Shepherd of the flock. The boy had known just a little bit about Jesus before, probably from a pious mother or from some playmates, but until now he had not "belonged."

We pray that even today he is still a sheep of God's pasture, living the life that leads to the heavenly Sheepfold!

A "BAD" BOY TURNED TO GOOD

Then there was Chuck, a friendly boy of about twelve years. He was as eager and lively in his growing up as any other normal boy. Unfortunately, he was being raised in a home that had no deep interest in religion, and so his sense of right and wrong was warped.

One evening in the company of his neighborhood friends, he joined in taunting a Chinese laundryman by tossing stones against his shop windows. It was a favorite trick of the boys because they knew that the man became very angry when they teased him.

This evening the boys once again played their trick, and the Chinese man lost his composure. He reached under his counter, pulled out a revolver, and began chasing the boys up a dark alley beside the shop. In his fury, he fired the gun blindly several times after the fleeing boys. One of the shots struck Chuck in the middle of his back, and he was seriously hurt.

An ambulance was called, and the boy was rushed to Emergency Hospital. A hasty examination prompted the physician in charge to call the nurses' station, and from there the request came for a Lutheran pastor to come quickly to visit the critically-injured boy.

When I arrived at the bedside about twenty minutes later, I found a very frightened youngster, awed by the scene of several doctors and nurses working swiftly and silently in the midst of intravenous tubes and blood transfusion apparatus, preparing the boy for surgery that might save his life.

The boy was conscious enough to sense what was going on. When I asked him if he knew what these people were doing, he answered, "They're trying to save my life." And that gave me an open door to enter to tell him about our Savior, who had bled and died to save our life from sin, death, and hell. Because Jesus died for us, God could now promise us forgiveness for all wrongs and a life with him in heaven that never ends. He said, "Yes," when I asked directly if he knew of and believed in that Jesus.

I found out later from an older brother that one of the lads in the "gang" had at times taken Chuck along to Sunday school. So the name of Jesus was not entirely new to him. But until this serious moment it never seemed to be important to know him better.

Then, back to the bed. The medical team stood aside for a moment as I spoke a fervent prayer that the Lord would guide the surgeon in helping Chuck. I also prayed that God would let his gracious will be done. Then Chuck again amazed me by joining faintly in repeating the Lord's Prayer. He had learned it from his friend.

Well, they put him on a cart and wheeled him off to surgery. For about five hours they worked without a break, but the gun shot had done so much damage internally that Chuck never returned from the operating room alive.

God had a reason for taking a twelve-year-old home. One reason was to spare Chuck from further evil influences that might destroy his soul forever. Another reason could have been to renew the interest of his family in the one thing needful, the Word of God. It alone can prepare anyone for the judgment and the life to come beyond the grave. We stressed this at the funeral services for little Chuck and were assured later that at least some of the members of the family had returned to active church life.

A tragedy? Of course, but also blessing came to one of the many lambs who had never really gotten close to the Great Shepherd's flock . . . until the Shepherd brought him home.

GROUP CONFIRMATION

The Children's Home has been mentioned earlier. Out of its large population, we garnered about twenty-five to thirty-five children each spring for confirmation. The children dutifully fulfilled their obligations in the classes that were much like any church class. And then would come the big day—confirmation!

The attendants at the home had a "sunshine fund" out of which they bought gifts for the children on special occasions. At confirmation the fund provided new white dresses for the girls and a new pair of pants and a white shirt and tie for the boys. Both got a new pair of shoes. This in itself reminded the class that they were having a very special day to remember for the rest of their lives.

However, the happy hearts and faces of the children were the product of the Holy Spirit. He had given them the gift of all gifts, their faith that they were children of their heavenly Father, who would lead them through the treacherous valleys and over the rugged hilltops of life.

Chapel services were always a joy, but Confirmation Day, with its special solemnity, was most uplifting. Prepared properly, the children were sincere in making their vows before the assembly and receiving their certificates. All were happy, in spite of the fact that seldom did any relative from the outside put in an appearance for the festivities.

The staff of the home allowed another special privilege that day. The class was seated at a special table in the dining hall for official personnel. The meal was planned with extra care, and the superintendent and other guests would eat with us. All in all, it was a festive day not easily forgotten. To this day, it happens that a confirmand of many years ago will call or stop at our home to exchange pleasantries and say "thank you" for what was done for them. One came from faraway Arizona, another from Florida.

May the Good Shepherd keep them faithful forever!

AN UNUSUAL WEDDING

Many of the children at the Home formed lasting friendships while there. Some of them married and lived happily with the children the Lord gave them. Their experience in the Home set a pattern that helped shape their future, and the Home's chapel remained the sentimental focus of their church life.

This brings to mind the story of Elaine, one of five siblings who had been deserted by their parents. Though all of them were nice children, Elaine was the type who was a bit more loving and motherly, and one who leaned more trustingly on the advice of older people.

At age sixteen she heard of her mother's residing in a large city about 100 miles away. Elaine established contact and was invited to visit the one she wanted to love so deeply because, after all, she had brought her into the world. Planning the trip was thrilling after years of isolation. Perhaps she might even be able to make her home with her mother!

Elaine went to the strange big city and suddenly felt "all grown up." It took only a few days after her warm welcome there to realize, however, that the mother was living a life of sin, and that she expected her daughter to engage in the same illicit relationships. Elaine was so disheartened and disillusioned that she used all but a few of her dollars to buy a train ticket to New York, "to get away as far as possible from such iniquity."

She was hungry and penniless when she got there, and as she walked aimlessly down one street after another, she came to a church. It was a Lutheran Church, and Elaine mustered up courage to enter it. She found the pastor, a kindly gentleman, who listened patiently to her sad story. When she told him about her connections in Milwaukee, he called us and made arrangements for her to return.

Back at the Home, Elaine became a helper in the superintendent's home and enrolled in a nurses' training course so that she might in the future help others as God had helped her. On completion of the course and while working in a hospital she met a young man, one who had also grown up at the Home. They fell in love and prepared to marry. How happy we all were for Elaine!

But now the practical problems arose. Where would Elaine get a dress and other fineries for the wedding? Where would the groom get a suit? Where could they have the wedding, the kind that we felt she deserved? Not because of, but in spite of our fretting, things fell into place easily. My wife offered her own wedding gown and veil from some years ago. It fit Elaine, and she was thrilled! A suit was found at modest cost for groom Elmer. And with the help of the superintendent, permission was granted to perform the ceremony at the altar both knew as the place where God had taught them to know their Shepherd-Savior Jesus. For the first time in the history of the local public institutions, a wedding was held in the chapel of the Children's Home!

The staff provided the extras like flowers, food, and drink for the reception. All the children were invited and had a good time. So touching and refreshing was the story, that the news media sent reporters and a camera crew to the event. Best of all in the memory, though, is the sincerity and devotional attitude of Elaine and Elmer as they repeated their vows before God. Following his leading, they were sure all would be well with them.

As they found employment the couple moved out of state. The first letter we received from them spoke of their gratitude and sense of belonging in their new church far away. They felt secure. The same loving Shepherd was there.

A TRACT ATTRACTS

Some of God's children are "born into the church." They come from a Christian home, are baptized as babies, and hear the Shepherd's voice from infancy on. Others may live their lives almost to the end before recognizing and following the voice. And some, in their old age, hear it in a strange manner.

A phone call summoned me one day to stop, at my convenience, at the home of an aged man. He had gotten my name from a tract he had brought home after a recent hospital stay.

When I arrived at the address that afternoon, I found this aged man and his sickly wife. Both were in their high eighties, living in a dingy one-room apartment in a rapidly decaying area of the city. Poverty was written all over the scene. Off in one corner of the room there was a cot on which the sick wife rested.

There was a larger bed in another corner, and in between a sofa that had seen better days. The rest of the room contained a hot plate for preparing meals, a small cooler, a sink, and a small cabinet for supplies. The bathroom was a shared room down the hallway. The linoleum on the floor was worn through the pattern to its base.

The man told me that while he had been a patient at the hospital he had heard me minister to another man in the ward, and what he heard kept coming back to his mind. Besides, he picked up the tract I had distributed, read it over and over, and later shared it with his ailing wife.

The tract spoke plainly of man's sin, God's justice and punishment, and mainly about God's forgiveness through the Lamb that was slain to set us free. Since the couple knew that it might not be long before they would meet their Judge, the tract had a tremendous effect on them, so much that they boldly decided to call me for further direction. Eternity was near, along with the appeal: "Come to me, all you who are weary and burdened, and I will give you rest"—an invitation and promise they could not ignore any longer. That rest and peace they now coveted for their aroused consciences. They wanted the assurance that it was theirs too, as God's gift to hopeless man.

Arrangements were made with a cooperative neighboring pastor to call on the couple. He did, often. After a period of instruction in Christian truth, he baptized and confirmed them in the presence of witnesses from his church. Thus they "joined the flock." A little tract had done its work as the calling card of the Good Shepherd. It had helped bring some of his "other sheep" to his fold.

A DESIRE FULFILLED

Speaking of the aged, what riches and encouragement we can find in their thoughts and actions! Someone has said, "An old person knows what it is like to be young, but a young person does not know what it means to be old." It is sound advice that the younger generations respect, honor, and heed the good counsel of their elders. This is also biblical doctrine.

Of course, the aged can make serious mistakes in judgment, especially in matters of Christian faith and life. They may set a bad example for the young when they fail to openly confess Jesus as Lord and Savior. But it is not always that they don't want to confess. A long list of circumstantial happenings may help to deter them and create the failings.

I was reminded of this while musing over a visit with a ninety-six-year-old grandmother, to whose side I had been called by a nurse at the hospital. She "just had to speak to a pastor."

This was her first trip to the hospital in many years, and she felt it might be her last. There was something on her heart that she wanted to share with a pastor, one whom she could trust as a representative of God. Weakly, but at length, she spoke that afternoon of her past life, her struggles for survival in financial reverses, her bitter tears shed over wayward family members, and also of the loneliness that was engulfing her in dark shadows growing ever longer toward evening.

Yet the real thing she wanted to talk about was her relationship to God and his Son Jesus, Savior of sinners. We were most surprised to hear her make a clear and very firm request for holy baptism. Oh yes, she assured me; she knew about God and her need for his promised pardon for sin. She believed that there was no other Redeemer beside Jesus Christ the crucified. She was sure there was no hope of heaven, without complete reliance on his merits. All this had come to her through reading the Bible and occasional attendance at church services. In her own way she had been listening to the voice of the Shepherd, while not really responding to it.

She well knew the Lord's words: "Whoever believes and is baptized will be saved." But not until now had she been able to make herself confess it all openly and sincerely. "Pastor, will you baptize me?"

After a brief review of our guilt before God and a reminder of the cleansing power of Jesus' blood, she was baptized in the presence of nurse witnesses. If we who were present could be happy, how the angels in heaven must have sung their "Te Deum" that day, as the Shepherd carried another sheep home on his shoulders rejoicing.

The happy but weary sheep lived for several weeks after that, but it was a different kind of life, much richer than anything she had known before. There was gratitude that only a Christian can know. There was satisfaction in the knowledge that her long, inexcusable procrastination had not ended in unstoppable misery.

PATIENCE IN WAITING

Sooner or later, all of us learn the lesson that it is not easy to grow old and weak. Eyesight dims, hearing becomes muffled, legs and arms ache and shake. A feeling of uselessness and helplessness becomes a daily unwelcome companion. It's bad enough when an aged person still has a family of sorts and a home, but when these heavy years must be lived among strangers in some large institution, life sometimes becomes almost unbearable.

Karl is now a little short of the century mark in years. His mind was clear and sharp as he related stories of his childhood and youth. The memories are not all good though, because his stepfather never was like a real father to him. He was not close to Karl, nor did he have any sympathy for his problems and pains.

In bygone years "spells" (epilepsy) were considered untreatable, except by custodial care in an asylum. When Karl was diagnosed, he soon found himself an inmate with two thousand others, young and old, who suffered from some kind of mental health impairment. Many years he spent in these depressing surroundings. But it really wasn't all that bad. Once one passed the adjustment period and forgot about anything resembling home—why, one could get along as one's stamina developed.

When his family gradually died out, Karl was a very lonely and confused individual, seeking some kind of redemption from his plight. Most helpful to him in setting his own way of life were the seeds that were sown in his mind and heart when he began to attend chapel services conducted by a Lutheran missionary pastor. He tells how he "sopped up" the kindliness of the pastor during many months of instruction in Christian doctrine, and he loves to recall the day of his confirmation when he pledged his allegiance to the Good Shepherd Jesus. Though before he had no one and nothing, he now possessed all. His Savior was his dearest Friend.

Over many years the seizures diminished and then ended entirely. But where "on the outside" would you place an aging man, definitely restricted in learning and the usual graces? Karl had always been industrious and a willing worker at any task assigned to him. He was friendly, dependable, and honest. He would tell you today, "That is the way it should be; that is pleasing to God."

The Shepherd found a way for his sheep. Jobs were plentiful as many men were serving in the armed forces during World War II. And a job was found for Karl! He became a houseman in a hospital that offered clean and cozy living quarters and meals to specified workers. Since Karl was highly recommended, he was one of the privileged ones. He knew it and tried to repay such kindness with his best efforts on the job.

It took several years of scrimping and saving, but he persevered in reaching his goal: buying a life contract in a home for aging. Here, among others of his faith, his happiness grew to new heights! Who would ever have imagined that his life would lead into such pleasant places! For all this, and even for the many hardships of his life, he daily thanks God for lavishly providing for him. This was truly a happy sheep of the fold.

Today, nearing the 100 mark in years, he still occupies his time in making things for others: scratch pads, holiday decorations, and other things that he sends to his few remaining friends. He also does some excellent weaving on the loom. Most people who see his work marvel at his artistry, and they remark about an unfailing central theme to all his work, the prominence of the Shepherd who came to mean so much to Karl.

As shadows fall, that Savior is his life and all. Karl can think of nothing finer than the day of his departure to life eternal. But he is willing to wait for the Shepherd's call. Jesus has never failed him. He will not fail him now.

DOESN'T ANYONE CARE?

One of the sheep that has run the whole gamut of ills from birth to the present day is Bertha, now in her sixties. She was born with serious physical defects that have kept her in a wheel-chair or in bed all her life. Yet she is a most cheerful person because her Shepherd found her and has remained with her through many trials.

Bertha, the lastborn in her family, is severely physically handicapped. She is not able to use her arms or legs, yet her mind is clear and sharp. She is totally dependent on the help others can give her.

Her mother died when Bertha was a little child, and her father was never able to care for her. Bereft of parents, with brothers and sisters scattered abroad, she has learned to live but for one thing: the fulfillment of her hope that one day her Shepherd will release her from the woes of this life and take her to heaven.

I met her when she was fifteen and had been placed in the county infirmary to live with hundreds of aged, dependent, and homeless men and women. And what a trying time in life it proved to be! She was unhappy, afraid of tomorrow. There was not much that anyone could do to ease her discomfort of body and mind.

But the Lord used those very circumstances to soften her heart and give her hope. We talked about the ravages of sin as displayed in her very body. We also talked about the bitterness that develops when we feel deprived of many things others may enjoy. But mainly, our conversations focused on Jesus, who came in human flesh to be our Brother; to suffer our deserved punishment and pains; to taste rejection even by those he loved; and finally to die on a cross, all for us! Though we still face sufferings in life, they are not punishments from an angry God but ways and means he uses to keep us in faith and bring us to the mansions of heaven.

Bertha quickly grasped the meaning of it all, and by the power of the convincing Word, she gave her heart and life to the Savior. She was confirmed in the faith and became an ardent worshiper and communicant.

As the years passed by, Bertha was transferred from one home to another, but always kept her contact with our ministry. And all through the times of various illnesses and crises, she has been served faithfully by our pastors. Every month she partakes of the sacrament of Communion, and whenever she is in a home where we conduct chapel worship, she is always present at the services. She is hopeful and of happy mind, a fruit of faith seldom found in one who has so constantly been in the refiner's fire. Each month she manages to put aside a share of her welfare payment so that she can bring a heartfelt gift to her Savior. What a lesson for us who are so richly blessed with health and great stores of this world's goods!

During Lent you will find her to be a solemn person, and on Good Friday she relives in thought the Savior's agonies. That is when she particularly desires the sacrament as a reassurance that her sins are covered by Jesus' blood. On one such Good Friday, a few years ago, she was exhilarated and joyful, even though she was usually deeply contemplative and of sad appearance. After I had ended our private Communion service, I asked why she appeared to be so light-hearted. Her reply was: "I've been thinking about the crucifixion all week. Good Friday is sad, but after that comes Easter Sunday when Jesus rose from his grave. He promised that we too will rise from our grave someday, and he will clothe us in a glorified and perfect body. For the first time then I will be able to use my arms and legs. I will be able to walk and talk plainly. I won't need people helping me, feeding me, dressing me, pushing my wheelchair, and putting me to bed. What a wonderful day is coming!"

I think we can understand her elation at the prospect of being a perfect sheep of the fold, enjoying forever the bliss of complete contentment.

POTTERS' FIELD

Hundreds upon hundreds of the Shepherd's sheep have been laid to rest to await the trumpet call to resurrection on the last day. In our families, we are happy when loving hands and hearts pay their final respects and solemnly tend the deceased. But it is not always so with the institutionalized. Society too often depersonalizes the individual who is hidden away from common contacts.

So it frequently happens that a forgotten or unwanted one finds a resting place in a "potters' field." Each large urban community has such a place for the burial of unclaimed bodies. And we have often used our potters' field to lay to rest the remains of infants whom we have baptized on their deathbed, youths who had been "discarded" by their parents, and mainly aged Christians without families or friends. Each grave is marked by a small brass plate with a number, and a record is kept in general administration offices.

Today, however, the potters' field has changed and is rarely used anymore. Public welfare policies now allow limited monies to be used for burial plots in private and commercial cemeteries. A modest casket and wood vault are provided, quite unlike the facilities of years ago. Then the caskets were of plywood with four large handles, unlined by any soft materials, and of hexagonal shape. The caskets and burial boxes were quickly hammered together by workers in the Infirmary carpenter shop whenever needed, and the "boss" acted as mortician.

A truck would serve as the hearse, and almost always there were but three people attending the burial: the pastor and two Infirmary workers. It was a cold and crude happening. "For we brought nothing into the world, and we can take nothing out of it."

But with the Spirit of God there in the Word and prayer, these burials were as grand as any in the world's largest cathedrals. At the great resurrection when Jesus comes again to judge all, these humble saints of God will stand regally before the King of heaven and earth. They will thank him and sing his praises for the gift more important than a burial place: the gift of life everlasting!

CONCLUSION

God has charged his church with the command: "Go into all the world and preach the good news to all creation." All men must hear the voice of the Good Shepherd in order for them to know the faith that saves from perdition.

By God's grace, you and I have been sanctified to bear the Master's image, and we have been consecrated to do his will. We are sowers of saving truth in the world of people, just sowers. We spread the seed but have no power to produce the harvest. Only God can let the sunshine and rain of his blessing bring the results he desires. Only he can produce faith; only he can preserve it. Only he can forgive our sins and give us eternal life.

With firm faith in his promises and aware of the urgency "do the work of him who sent me. Night is coming, when no one can work." We accept the honor of being his coworkers in holding the door to heaven open for all. Our greatest satisfaction in life comes from remembering the things he lets us do for others in his name.

For others? Surely our hearts must be touched by the many bruised, beaten, sick, wandering, erring, and rebelling sheep included in the Shepherd's concerns. Many of them we will find in institutions of every kind throughout the world. In our nation alone, statisticians have set their number at more than thirty-three million! What a privilege is accorded us in serving these "other sheep"! What joy will echo throughout heaven when we meet the rescued and restored sheep in the eternal fold one day!

Gradually, all of us might become impersonal numbers on Social Security cards. Medicare and Medicaid may hide us under reams of bureaucratic paperwork. But man will remain man, by nature a lost sheep in need of a shepherd. As our population ages, probably more and more of the sheep will be herded into nursing and convalescent homes, into public housing projects, into prisons. Will there be shepherds to serve their never-diminishing spiritual needs?

The stories in this book, we pray, may whet the appetite of many able Christians to practice true charity toward their unfortunate and needy fellow pilgrims along life's road. Actually, the investments of talent, time, and tangible assets are minimal compared with the rich spiritual dividends paid by the Good Shepherd.

There is a story told about a spinster in a New England town who was sitting and rocking comfortably before her fireplace on a blizzardy, cold night. She had never had much to do with neighbors and townspeople but was content to live only for herself. On this night, just before bedtime, she thought she heard a noise outside the door. It sounded like the weak wailing of an infant in distress. When the howling winds would temporarily subside, she heard the wail again and again. Finally she unlatched the door and opened it. There on her doorstep was an abandoned child wrapped warmly in a bundle of blankets.

There were no social service agencies in those days and no emergency hospital facilities. What was she to do but take the infant into her home and care for it at least until morning? She did that. She gave the baby warm milk, dry clothes.

To lull it to sleep, she sat down before the fire and rocked in her chair.

She fell asleep, and then she dreamed a dream. She was on the road to heaven. Rough and narrow was the path, bumpy and rocky, with brambles and branches and thorns tearing away at her. She stumbled and fell often, painfully bruising herself. It didn't help the situation to be carrying the baby.

Once, when she fell, she pulled back the blanket and looked into the baby's tiny face. Something happened to her at that moment, and the ice around her heart began to thaw. She loved this child who needed her so much. And all the coldness and self-interest that had filled the dark corners of her heart before disappeared. One thing only mattered—to protect the helpless one and carry it with her to heaven.

The road was all at once smooth and broad, and invisible arms seemed to lift and carry her onward to her goal. Then she saw the end of the road and the mansions of eternity filled with the happy ones who had entered there before. As she stood gazing and marveling, an angel came out of the door and approached her. Without speaking a word his finger wrote on her brow, no longer showing signs of weariness or bitterness or selfishness, the one word: "Whatever."

[31] "When the Son of Man comes in his glory, and all the angels with him, he will sit on his throne in heavenly glory. [32] All the nations will be gathered before him, and he will separate the people one from another as a shepherd separates the sheep from the goats. [33] He will put the sheep on his right and the goats on his left.

[34] "Then the King will say to those on his right, 'Come, you who are blessed by my Father; take your inheritance, the kingdom prepared for you since the creation of the world. [35] For I was hungry and you gave me something to eat, I was thirsty and you gave me something to drink, I was a stranger and you invited me in, [36] I needed clothes and you clothed me, I was sick and you looked after me, I was in prison and you came to visit me.'

[37] "Then the righteous will answer him, 'Lord, when did we see you hungry and feed you, or thirsty and give you something to drink? [38] When did we see you a stranger and invite you in or needing clothes and clothe you? [39] When did we see you sick or in prison and go to visit you?'

[40] "The King will reply, 'I tell you the truth, whatever you did for one of the least of these brothers of mine, you did for me.'" Matthew 25:31–40 (NIV84)